EYE AND VISION RESEARCH DEVELOPMENTS

CATARACTS AND CATARACT SURGERY

TYPES, RISK FACTORS, AND TREATMENT OPTIONS

EYE AND VISION RESEARCH DEVELOPMENTS

Additional books in this series can be found on Nova's website under the Series tab.

Additional e-books in this series can be found on Nova's website under the e-book tab.

EYE AND VISION RESEARCH DEVELOPMENTS

CATARACTS AND CATARACT SURGERY

TYPES, RISK FACTORS, AND TREATMENT OPTIONS

DIDIER NAVARRO
EDITOR

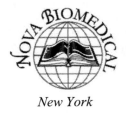

New York

Copyright © 2013 by Nova Science Publishers, Inc.

All rights reserved. No part of this book may be reproduced, stored in a retrieval system or transmitted in any form or by any means: electronic, electrostatic, magnetic, tape, mechanical photocopying, recording or otherwise without the written permission of the Publisher.

For permission to use material from this book please contact us:
Telephone 631-231-7269; Fax 631-231-8175
Web Site: http://www.novapublishers.com

NOTICE TO THE READER

The Publisher has taken reasonable care in the preparation of this book, but makes no expressed or implied warranty of any kind and assumes no responsibility for any errors or omissions. No liability is assumed for incidental or consequential damages in connection with or arising out of information contained in this book. The Publisher shall not be liable for any special, consequential, or exemplary damages resulting, in whole or in part, from the readers' use of, or reliance upon, this material. Any parts of this book based on government reports are so indicated and copyright is claimed for those parts to the extent applicable to compilations of such works.

Independent verification should be sought for any data, advice or recommendations contained in this book. In addition, no responsibility is assumed by the publisher for any injury and/or damage to persons or property arising from any methods, products, instructions, ideas or otherwise contained in this publication.

This publication is designed to provide accurate and authoritative information with regard to the subject matter covered herein. It is sold with the clear understanding that the Publisher is not engaged in rendering legal or any other professional services. If legal or any other expert assistance is required, the services of a competent person should be sought. FROM A DECLARATION OF PARTICIPANTS JOINTLY ADOPTED BY A COMMITTEE OF THE AMERICAN BAR ASSOCIATION AND A COMMITTEE OF PUBLISHERS.

Additional color graphics may be available in the e-book version of this book.

Library of Congress Cataloging-in-Publication Data

ISBN: 978-1-62808-400-9
Library of Congress Control Number: 2013942944

Published by Nova Science Publishers, Inc. † New York

Contents

Preface		vii
Chapter I	Clinical Techniques to Assess the Visual and Optical Performance of Intraocular Lenses: A Review *Amit Navin Jinabhai, Graeme Young,* *Lee Anthony Hall and James Stuart Wolffsohn*	1
Chapter II	Cataracts: Epidemiology, Morphology, Types and Risk Factors *Dieudonne Kaimbo Wa Kaimbo*	59
Chapter III	A Practical Guide to the Management of Intraoperative Floppy Iris Syndrome (IFIS) *Allan Storr-Paulsen*	111
Chapter IV	A Comparison of Safety and Visual Improvement of Phacoemulsification with Sutureless Single-Port 25-Gauge Vitrectomy versus Phacoemulsicátion Alone for Eyes with Extremely Shallow Anterior Chambers *Hiroshi Kobayashi*	123
Chapter V	Teaching and Learning Cataract Surgery *Sandra M. Johnson and Eric Areiter*	137
Chapter VI	Phacolytic Glaucoma *Kayoung Yi and Teresa C. Chen*	145
Index		153

Preface

This book discusses the types, risk factors, treatment options and potential complications of cataracts and cataract surgery. Topics include the clinical techniques used to assess the visual and optical performance of intraocular lenses; the epidemiology and morphology of cataracts; a practical guide to the management of intraoperative floppy iris syndrome (IFIS); a comparison of safety and visual improvement of phacoemulsification with sutureless single-port 25-gauge vitrectomy versus phacoemulsification alone for eyes with extremely shallow anterior chamber; teaching and learning cataract surgery; and phacolytic glaucoma.

Chapter I - A number of clinical techniques are available to assess the visual and optical performance of the eye. This report aims to review the advantages and limitations of techniques used in previous studies of patients implanted with intraocular lenses (IOLs), whose designs are ever increasing in optical complexity. Although useful, *in-vitro* measurements of IOL optical quality cannot account for the wide range of biological variation in ocular anatomy and corneal optics, which will impact on the visual outcome achieved. This further highlights the need for a standardised series of visual performance tests that can be applied to a wide range of IOL designs. The conclusions of this report intend to assist researchers in developing a comprehensive series of investigations to evaluate IOL performance. Repeatable and reproducible *in-vivo* assessments of visual and optical performance are desirable to further develop IOL concepts and designs, in the hope of improving current post-operative visual satisfaction.

Chapter II - Cataract is the leading cause of blindness (defined as visual acuity less than 20/400) worldwide and is responsible for approximately 50% of the estimated 40 million cases of blindness in the developing world. In the next 20 years there will be doubling of cataract visual morbidity. Oxidation of lens proteins and mitochondrial function are key factors in cataract pathogenesis. This chapter focuses on epidemiology, morphology and different types of cataracts. The chapter also presents a comprehensive overview of specific and general cataract risk factors. Contents based on recent findings published in the medical literature and will reflect the most advanced achievements in current clinical and experimental research on cataracts.

Chapter III - Intraocular floppy iris syndrome (IFIS) observed during cataract surgery includes fluttering and billowing of the iris, a propensity for iris prolapse though incisions, and constriction of the pupil leading to higher rates of complications. Although IFIS may have a multifactorial background, it is most often associated with the chronic use of systemic sympathetic α-1 AR antagonists, and tamsulosin in particular. But many other drugs, and even alternative medicine have been reported to cause a floppy iris. Management of IFIS includes preoperative precautions such as thorough questioning of the medical history, and α-1a antagonists in particular. Moreover, we propose a surgical strategy including the use of a high viscous viscoelastic, the use of pupil expansions rings, and to keep phenylephrine ready for intracameral injection in case of a progressive pupil constriction during surgery.

Chapter IV – Purpose: To compare the visual improvement and safety of phacoemulsication with suturelss transconjunctival single-port 25-gauge vitrectomy and phacoemulsication for eyes with extremely shallow anterior chamber.

Methods: Forty patients with 2.5 mm or less of the anterior chamber depth who were scheduled to undergo phacoemulsification and intraocular lens implantation were studied. Eyes were assigned randomly to either phacoemulsication with 25-gauge vitrectomy or phacoemulsication alone. Patients were followed-up for 6 months and the incidence of intra- and postoperative complications was compared.

Results: Mean anterior chamber depth was 2.19 ± 0.22 mm in the phacoemulsication with vitrectomy group and 2.17 ± 0.25 mm in the phacoemulsication alone group ($P = 0.8$). There was no significant difference in the mean best-corrected visual acuity between the groups at any time point before and after surgery. neal endothelial cell density at baseline and at 6 months postoperatively was $2420\pm360/mm^2$ and $2282\pm 3331/mm^2$ in the phacoemulsication with vitrectomy group and $2436\pm313/mm^2$ and $2248\pm335/mm^2$ in the phacoemulsication alone group, respectively. The phacoemulsication alone group showed a loss of 7.9 ± 3.0 % at 6 months in the change of corneal endothelium cell density, which was significantly greater than that of the phacoemusication with vitrectomy group (P = 0.0057) Complications included two cases (10 %) of continuous curvilinear capsulorhexis tear in the phacoemulsication alone group, whereas two cases (8%) of zonular dehiscence occurred in each group.

Chapter V - Introduction: The most common procedure done by ophthalmology resident surgeons is cataract surgery. This is the back bone procedure for their training and aims at treating the most common cause of blindness in the world.

Methods: This chapter is based on a literature review of resident cataract surgery and resident surgery in general.

Results: Information is available on teaching the phacoemulsification techniques of cataract surgery and regarding resident outcomes for this.

Conclusion: An awareness of the methods, issues and outcomes for resident cataract surgeons can serve to enhance the practice. More information is needed regarding teaching the technique of small incision extra capsular cataract surgery.

Chapter VI - Phacolytic glaucoma is a rare complication of an advanced cataract. Phacolytic glaucoma is usually an acute open angle glaucoma that develops from blockade of the trabecular meshwork by leakage of lens protein from a mature or hypermature cataract. Even though the incidence of phacolytic glaucoma is decreasing due to the availability of earlier cataract surgery, it is still in the differential diagnosis of acute elevated intraocular pressure (IOP) in patients with a dense cataract. Although phacolytic glaucoma usually occurs with a mature or hypermature cataract, it less is associated with focal liquefaction of an immature cataract. Slit lamp examination reveals high eye pressures with corneal edema, mid-dilated pupil, intense flare and large cells, and/or hyperrefringent particles. Keratic precipitates are not typically present. Initial treatment is focused on lowering the IOP with glaucoma medications and decreasing the inflammation with topical steroids. Definitive treatment is cataract extraction. The prognosis of phacolytic glaucoma is usually excellent, but delayed treatment may cause permanent damage to the optic nerve and/or cornea, resulting in a poor outcome. If IOP elevation persists after cataract surgery, additional medical and/or surgical management may be required.

In: Cataracts and Cataract Surgery
Editor: Didier Navarro

ISBN: 978-1-62808-400-9
© 2013 Nova Science Publishers, Inc.

Chapter I

Clinical Techniques to Assess the Visual and Optical Performance of Intraocular Lenses: A Review

Amit Navin Jinabhai,[1,2,3] *Graeme Young,*[1,2]
Lee Anthony Hall[1,2] *and James Stuart Wolffsohn*[1,2]

[1]Ophthalmic Research Group; School of Life and Health Sciences, Aston University, Birmingham, UK
[2]Visioncare Research Ltd., Farnham, Surrey, UK
[3]Faculty of Life Sciences, The University of Manchester, Manchester, UK

Abstract

A number of clinical techniques are available to assess the visual and optical performance of the eye. This report aims to review the advantages and limitations of techniques used in previous studies of patients implanted with intraocular lenses (IOLs), whose designs are ever increasing in optical complexity. Although useful, *in-vitro* measurements of IOL optical quality cannot account for the wide range of biological variation in ocular anatomy and corneal optics, which will impact on the visual outcome achieved. This further highlights the need for a standardised series of visual performance tests that can be applied to a wide range of IOL designs. The conclusions of this report intend to assist researchers in developing a comprehensive series of investigations to evaluate IOL performance. Repeatable and reproducible *in-vivo* assessments of visual and optical performance are desirable to further develop IOL concepts and designs, in the hope of improving current post-operative visual satisfaction.

1. Introduction

A perplexing variety of techniques is available to assess the visual and optical performance of the eye. This report aims to review the possible advantages and disadvantages of methods used in previous studies of patients implanted with intraocular lenses (IOLs), whose designs are increasing in optical complexity. Repeatable and reproducible *in-vivo* evaluations of visual and optical performance would prove useful in developing better IOL designs and concepts, to improve upon current levels of post-operative visual satisfaction. Although useful, *in-vitro* measurements of IOL optical quality cannot account for the wide range of biological variation in ocular anatomy (e.g. anterior chamber depth and axial length) and corneal optics, which will impact on the visual outcome achieved for each patient. This further highlights the need for a standardised series of clinical visual performance tests that can be applied to a wide range of different IOL types. The conclusions of this report intend to support the design of a comprehensive series of tests to evaluate IOL performance.

2. Visual Acuity

Most studies concerning IOL visual performance have used logMAR-principle letter charts, such as the Bailey-Lovie, [1] Regan letter [2] or Early Treatment of Diabetic Retinopathy Study (ETDRS), charts. [3] Compared to Snellen acuity, LogMAR letter charts offer the advantages of:

- Simple numerical results facilitating statistical analyses,
- An equal number of letters per line (reduces the risk of guessing correctly), and
- A regular logarithmic progression of letter size between lines (non-truncated).

In addition to high-contrast acuity letters, logMAR letter charts are also available at lower levels of contrast. [4, 5]

Key factors for measuring visual acuity (VA) include the illuminance/luminance of the target letters and the physical distance of the chart from the patient. [6] To ensure measurements are consistent for multi-site collaborative studies, it is imperative that these factors are kept as similar as possible at each site. Furthermore, other reports have demonstrated the importance of standardising the type of letter chart and scoring system used between sites to avoid measurement variations due to subtle differences amongst different logMAR chart designs. [7, 8] The instrument currently considered by the National Eye Institute (NEI) as the 'gold standard' for clinical acuity measurement is the ETDRS chart. [9, 10] The chart features Sloan optotypes designed to be comparable to Landolt's broken rings in terms of recognition difficulty. [11] Sloan letters include the characters C, D, K, H, N, Z, R, S, V and O, designed using 5 x 5-sized non-serif optotypes. The ETDRS chart comprises 14 lines (ranging from +1.00 to -0.30 log units in size), each with 5 letters when used at a distance of 4 m.

The recommended letter chart luminance for VA measurements varies between different countries; e.g. in the United States the recommended luminance is 85 cd/m^2, whereas in the United Kingdom, it is 120 cd/m^2 and 300 cd/m^2 in Germany. These differences between countries further highlight the importance of standardising measurement conditions between different investigational sites. Furthermore, if the letter chart luminance and room illumination levels become altered between repeated measurements of VA, for any given subject, such variations may cause alterations in the subject's pupil diameter and, therefore, higher-order aberrations, perhaps impacting on the visual performance achieved.

An even wider variety of reading charts is available to record near visual performance. [12] These include the MNRead (Minnesota Near Reading) acuity chart (Lighthouse Low Vision Products, NY, US); the Jaeger reading chart (Western Ophthalmics Corp., WA, US); the Birkhauser reading charts (Scalae Typographicae Birkhaeuseri, Birkhauser Verlag, Basel, Switzerland); the logMAR Lighthouse Near Visual Acuity Test (Lighthouse International, NY, US); the logMAR ETDRS near visual acuity chart (Precision Vision, IL, US); the Rosenbaum Nearvision card (Western Ophthalmics Corp.) and the logMAR Holladay contrast acuity test (Stereo Optical, IL, US). The latter four instruments are designed with single, uppercase optotypes only, whereas other charts use words and sentences with a mixture of both uppercase and lowercase letters. In contrast, the Practical Near Acuity Chart (PNAC) (Aston,

Birmingham, UK) and the Bailey-Lovie near chart (Sussex Vision International, Sussex, UK) use words and sentences containing lowercase letters only. Compared to the Bailey-Lovie near chart, the PNAC uses a fixed number of words per line (three) enabling quick measurements of near acuity, particularly for patients with visual impairment. [13] Unlike for distance VA measurements, word optotype targets allow a more realistic assessment of near visual performance compared to single letters. [14] However, word optotypes tend to yield poorer visual acuities compared to letter optotypes, [12, 15] perhaps as a result of contour interactions. [16] As with distance VA, near chart designs should be based on a logarithmic progression scale. The Jaeger near vision charts have been found to show inconsistent letter sizes for the same point size, [17] and coupled with their non-standard acuity level separation, this makes them a poor choice for evaluating near vision, despite the dominance of this instruments uses in previous clinical studies. Table 1 summarises the range of vision charts available for measuring visual acuity and functional reading ability.

Near logMAR letter charts are also available at low-contrast levels, with some authors suggesting that both high-contrast and low-contrast visual acuities should be measured under both photopic and mesopic lighting conditions in order to fully evaluate the level of visual performance achieved with a given IOL. [18-20]

The use of computerised software and display screens to measure VA has grown in popularity; examples of devices typically used in clinical practice include the electronic Thomson Vision Chart (Thomson Software Solutions, Hertfordshire, UK), [21] the COMPlog system (Medisoft; Leeds, UK) [22] and the Thomson Vision Toolbox application for the Apple iPad/iPhone (Apple Inc. California, US). [23] These platforms offer several advantages, including saving space within the consulting room (several charts can be presented with one device), allowing more accurate control of letter chart luminance, rapid presentation of high- and low-contrast optotypes and rapid target optotype randomisation. Interactive devices such as the iPad/iPhone can be used to improve data recording accuracy and reduce testing times, as these devices allow subjects to tap on their threshold optotypes. The device's computer can also be used to time the subject whilst reading and to analyse their data after completing the measurements.

Both Beck et al. [24] and Laidlaw et al. [22] have demonstrated equivalent repeatability between high-contrast VA measurements made with electronic ETDRS (e-ETDRS) and printed ETDRS charts in adults. [25] Similar findings have also been reported in children. [26] Likewise, Shah et al. [27] have shown comparable repeatability between VA measurements made with electronic and printed Kay's picture cards in both adults and children. Compared to traditional printed charts, electronic charts offer the advantage of improved standardisation across multiple sites. [24, 26] Originally, electronic test charts were presented on cathode ray tube (CRT) display screens; however, these devices tended to be bulky and induced unwanted flicker. Liquid crystal display (LCD) screens offer some advantages as they produce simultaneous high-contrast and high-luminance displays; are easily wall-mountable; are less susceptible to reflections from ambient lighting; use less energy and are aesthetically attractive. Some authors have reported a subjective preference of LCD over CRT screens for visual tasks; [28, 29] however, others have reported that LCD displays generate inferior low-contrast targets compared to CRT screens. [30-32] Some reports have also demonstrated slower visual search/recognition [33] and visually evoked potential (VEP) response times [30, 34] with LCD screens compared to with CRT screens; although increasing the contrast ratio and refresh rate may be helpful to overcome these issues. [28, 29] Overall, these contradictory findings suggest that more research is required to determine the influence of screen type on factors such as visual performance, visual fatigue and reaction time. [35]

Table 1. A summary of different vision charts available for measuring visual acuity and functional reading ability

Test	Description	Outcome measure
Snellen chart *Regan charts* *Bailey-Lovie chart* *Early treatment diabetic retinopathy study (ETDRS) chart*	Single, uppercase optotypes to measure logMAR visual acuity	High-contrast distance acuity (Regan, Bailey-Lovie and ETDRS charts are also available in low-contrast formats)
Jaeger reading chart *Birkhauser reading chart*	Words and sentences to measure near visual acuity (both with non-logarithmic progression)	High-contrast near acuity

Table 1. (Continued)

Test	Description	Outcome measure
Rosenbaum Nearvision Card *LogMAR Lighthouse Near Visual Acuity Chart* *LogMAR Holladay Contrast Acuity Test* *LogMAR ETDRS Near Chart*	Single, uppercase optotypes to measure near visual acuity (only the Rosenbaum card does not use a logarithmic progression between targets)	High-contrast near acuity (the LogMAR Holladay Contrast Acuity Test presents low-contrast targets)
Bailey-Lovie Near Chart	Lowercase, unrelated words with logarithmic progression	High-contrast near acuity (Also can be used to measure acuity reserve in low-vision patients)
Practical Near Acuity Chart (PNAC)	Words and sentences (three words per line) to measure near visual acuity. All words are lowercase and show a logarithmic progression.	High-contrast near acuity Reading speed (in words per minute) and fluency
Zeiss Near Vision Test Chart	Long text passages of approximately 830 characters in length (with logarithmic progression). Available in four languages for measuring reading ability.	Reading speed (in characters per minute)
Minnesota Near Reading (MNRead) Chart *Radner Reading Chart*	Words and sentences, (with logarithmic progression) to measure near visual acuity and functional reading ability.	High-contrast near acuity Maximum reading speed (in words per minute) Critical print size

3. Contrast Sensitivity

Like VA, contrast sensitivity describes visual performance under a limited set of conditions governed by factors such as the target's luminance, the selected testing distance and the subject's pupil size. Oshika et al. [36] have also demonstrated that contrast sensitivity is significantly correlated with ocular coma aberrations, which tend to increase in magnitude with increasing pupil diameter. [37-39] Various methods of recording contrast sensitivity have been reported, as it is widely accepted that a measurement of VA alone does not fully represent the visual disability induced by cataract. [40] Classically, the Pelli-Robson chart was used in most early IOL studies. [41, 42] However, a major limitation of this instrument is that all the optotypes are of the same size (spatial frequency); hence this methodology only evaluates a small element of the complete human contrast sensitivity function. [36, 43] Other tests, such as the Functional Acuity Contrast Test (FACT) chart (Vision Sciences Research Corp.; Walnut Creek, CA, US) [44, 45] and the CSV-1000E (Vector Vision, Greenville; OH, US) [46-48] have been selected in more recent investigations. Both these tests are based on the original Vistech Contrast Test System (Vistech Consultants Inc.; OH, US). [49] The FACT chart uses a forced-choice method and presents sine-wave gratings of 5 spatial frequencies (from 1.5 to 18 cycles/degree) at 9 different levels of contrast (from 0.5 % to 25 % contrast). The patient is asked to report the last grating they can see for each horizontal row (spatial frequency) and its orientation, as either right, up or left. The last correct grating seen for each spatial frequency is then plotted on a contrast sensitivity curve using specialised software (Eye View Functional Analysis Software; Vision Sciences Research Corp.). In addition, the FACT chart can be used to measure contrast sensitivity at two different controlled luminance levels: mesopic (6 cd/m^2) and photopic (85 cd/m^2). The chart is currently available for use at both distance and near.

The CSV-1000E test also uses a forced-choice methodology. The instrument features a series of photocells to monitor and calibrate luminance to 85 cd/m^2. At the testing distance of 2.5 metres, the chart displays sine-wave gratings at spatial frequencies of 3, 6, 12, and 18 cycles/degree, each on a separate row. Each row presents 17 circular patches (each 1.5 inches in diameter), the first presents a grating with high contrast for demonstration. The remaining patches are arranged into 8 columns along each row, decreasing in contrast from left to right. In each column, one grating is displayed in either the upper or lower patch, whereas the other patch is isoluminant (appears blank). Patients must identify which patch displays the grating (either top or bottom of the column) whilst viewing across each row. Subjects are encouraged to guess if a grating is at least partially visible; however, if no gratings are seen the response should be 'both blank'. The contrast level of the last correct response is recorded as the threshold value. As the potential to randomly guess the correct answer is high (one in two), measurements may become significantly distorted, perhaps overestimating visual performance. Nonetheless, the CSV-1000E device is designed with built-in glare sources (white LEDs) allowing contrast sensitivity measurement under glared conditions. [48] The Brightness Acuity Tester (BAT; model 1000, Marco Ophthalmic Inc. Jacksonville, FL, US) has also been used to create glare whilst measuring contrast sensitivity for patients implanted with multifocal IOLs. [50] However, this method tends to give inaccurate predictions of disability glare when using the device's high-intensity setting. [51, 52] Figure 1 displays the characteristics of various methods of assessing contrast sensitivity and the different parts of the contrast sensitivity function they encompass.

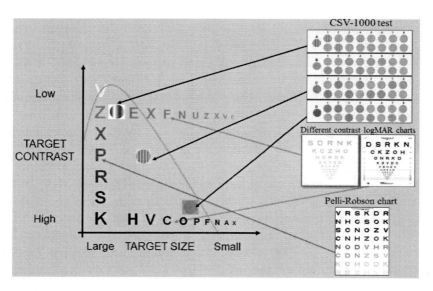

Figure 1. The contrast sensitivity function (CSF) curve demonstrating areas of the CSF assessed by different test methods.

Forced-choice contrast sensitivity tests, using sine-wave gratings, show poor repeatability in young healthy subjects, as well as cataract and post-LASIK patients. [53-55] Other reports have demonstrated 'ceiling' effects in young subjects and post-LASIK eyes [54, 56] and 'floor' effects in patients with cataract. [40, 56] This poor repeatability is likely due to the number of trials used; ideally, forced-choice tests should be performed with several repeated trials, as fewer trials typically show variable results. [57, 58] Additionally, forced-choice tests are prone to 'guessing' errors, e.g; with the FACT test, the subject has a one in three chance of correctly identifying the grating. Furthermore, forced-choice tests usually require longer testing times, [59] perhaps reducing the subject's concentration levels.

Given the aforementioned limitations, a simpler and faster method of assessing contrast sensitivity over a range of different distances is desirable. To date, most reports evaluating contrast sensitivity for patients implanted with IOLs have compared measurements between eyes implanted with multifocal and monofocal IOLs, [60-63] or have analysed the differences in contrast sensitivity between eyes implanted with aspheric and spherical IOLs. [47, 64-66]

4. Functional Reading Ability

In addition to near VA, near visual performance may also be evaluated through functional reading ability. Several reports have proposed that functional reading speed [67-69] and critical print size [70-73] should be used to evaluate visual performance for patients implanted with presbyopia-correcting IOLs. Particularly as it is widely accepted that patients with poorer near vision often require letters that are two (or more) times larger than their threshold acuity to achieve their maximum reading speed. [74]

Various metrics can be evaluated while assessing functional reading ability including:

1. Reading acuity (logMAR): the smallest print that can be read accurately without making significant errors. This measure is similar to distance VA, except that reading acuity is based on structured sentences rather than individual letters.
2. Maximum Reading Speed or MRS (in either words or characters per minute): Reading speed is usually determined for each sentence on the chart as the number of words read correctly, divided by the time taken to read the sentence. Therefore, in theory, the MRS is the reading speed with print larger than the critical print size, so that the subject's reading speed is not limited by the size of the print. Different approaches include averaging the supra-threshold reading speed

across multiple acuities [75, 76] and selecting the maximum reading speed achieved across supra-threshold acuities. [77]

3. Critical print size or CPS (logMAR): the smallest print at which the subject can read without a reduction in reading speed, hence, this is usually larger in size than the threshold reading VA. The CPS can be determined by observation of a plot of reading speed (ordinate) versus print size (abscissa). As the print size reduces, the reading speed falls outside of a defined confidence interval, or below a percentage of the supra-threshold reading speed. [76] The CPS can also be determined through mathematical curve fitting (exponential decay function). [78]

Whittaker and Lovie-Kitchin [79] suggested that a reading speed of at least 80 words per minute (wpm) is required for comfortable recreational reading. However, it is expected that reading speed will be unique for each person and is likely to be dependent on the subject's intellectual level, comprehension and motivation, [80] as well as other factors aside from visual clarity. Therefore, the complexity of the words and sentences used in the chart's design are also likely to influence reading speed. To overcome these issues, it has been proposed that the ideal instrument should use unrelated words (although this may appear to lack realism for the patient) and sentences of approximately equal legibility and syntactic complexity to minimise variability between sentences of different acuities. [14, 73, 80] Similarly, to account for potential differences in crowding/contour interactions, it is desirable to have an equal number of characters, spaces and words on each test line. [81] Test charts typically used to evaluate functional reading for patients with presbyopia-correcting IOLs include the Minnesota low-vision reading test (MNRead) chart (Lighthouse International, NY, US), [80] and the Radner chart (Precision Vision; La Salle, IL, US). [73]

Although both the MNRead and Radner test charts have been shown to provide repeatable [74, 75] and reliable results, [82] there are some limitations. For example, both charts are designed to be used at a recommended working distance of 40 cm only, rather than at the subject's own, habitual working distance. The charts also use short sentences with only a limited number of words on each line, therefore, any reading hesitation or timing error results in a large difference in the calculated reading speed.

Hahn et al. [83] developed an alternative reading chart, designed with longer texts of an equal length of 830 ± 2 characters (Zeiss Near Vision Test Chart; Cal Zeiss Meditec, Jena, Germany), which is available in four languages. Here, the number of characters is used to measure reading speed (in characters per minute) rather than the number of words, since the length of words can vary considerably between different languages. The charts have previously been adopted for measuring reading speed, [84] but not yet in studies of patients implanted with IOLs.

In addition to the metrics and measurements described above, Hutz and co-workers [68] have proposed measuring reading acuity and reading speed under different illumination conditions to elucidate differences in visual performance between different presbyopia-correcting IOLs. Such a methodology can also be coupled with measurements using medium-contrast and low-contrast targets to obtain a broader knowledge of the visual performance likely to be achieved under a range of different viewing conditions.

5. Assessment of Accommodation

Accommodation is defined as a dioptric change in the eye's power whilst focussing on a near object, resulting in a myopic refractive shift. [85] In a young phakic eye, the accommodative optical change is attributable to an increase in the power of the crystalline lens due to alterations in lens surface curvatures. [86-88] For pseudophakic patients fitted with presbyopia-correcting IOLs, the mechanism used to provide useful vision over a range of different distances varies depending on the lens platform. Currently commercialised, accommodating IOLs are based on two fundamental principles. Firstly, using a single optic design which moves anteriorly secondary to ciliary muscle contraction; such as the BioComfold IOL (*Morcher*, Stuttgart, Germany), Tek-Clear IOL (Tekia Inc. Irvine, CA, US), Kellan Tetraflex KH-3500 IOL (Lenstec, St Petersburg, FL, US), the Crystalens AO IOL (Bausch & Lomb, Rochester, NY, US) and the 1CU IOL (HumanOptics AG, Erlangen, Germany). The alternative method features a dual-optic design (Synchrony IOL; Abbott Medical Optics, San Clara, US), with a mobile positive lens (positioned anteriorly) and a stationary negative lens (positioned posteriorly). As the ciliary body contracts, the two lenses move further apart, using spring-loaded haptics, causing an increase in magnification and accommodation.

5.1. Subjective Measurement of Accommodation

5.1.1. Defocus Curves

Defocus curves are used to evaluate the subjective range of clear vision achieved with presbyopia-correcting IOLs; a schematic example is shown in Figure 2. Although defocus curves can be measured with targets placed at a range of distances in front of the eye, [89-92] this method is time consuming; furthermore, it is difficult to control for target size and luminance. Instead, the patient is usually first corrected for distance vision; subsequently their VA is then measured whilst viewing a distance letter chart (typically at 6 m) with lenses of negative (increasing the accommodative demand) and positive power (which should reduce VA if the distance refraction is optimal, allowing more precise curve-fitting) placed in front of the eye. Some studies have used a near rather than a distance letter chart; however, this seems to lead to a distorted defocus curve appearance. [93-95]

A wide variety of lens power ranges have been proposed to derive defocus curves when evaluating visual performance achieved with presbyopia-correcting IOLs. These vary between +6.00 to -6.00 D for multifocal IOLs, [96, 97] to +0.50 to -3.00 D for accommodating IOLs. [98, 99] Virtually all studies use 0.50 D-steps, but the usefulness of this increment size has not been confirmed. Polynomial curve-fitting can then be used to generate a range of metrics from the defocus curve (e.g. the area under the curve) which may enable differentiation between different presbyopia-correcting IOLs. [100-102]

The defocus induced by negative lenses is typically overcome by the accommodative element of the presbyopia-correcting IOL, or the patient's own accommodative ability if the patient under investigation is pre-presbyopic. Although defocus curves have been widely used to investigate the visual performance of presbyopia-correcting IOLs, several factors need to be considered while using this technique, such as monocular vs. binocular measurements, letter/lens randomisation, background illumination and target contrast. Measuring defocus curves binocularly, rather than monocularly, can better simulate most day-to-day visual tasks. Equally, binocular measurements are needed to assess 'mix-and-match' presbyopia-correcting options, such as monofocal IOLs fitted to achieve mono-vision, [103, 104] bifocal IOLs, [90, 105] multifocal IOLs [68, 106] or a combination of multifocal and monofocal IOLs. [107]

Gupta and co-workers [108] have demonstrated that it is important to consider randomisation of the defocus lenses, the test letters, or both, to overcome learning effects in younger subjects. The effects of learning could result in an overestimation of visual performance at different distances.

Changes in pupil size can affect the results of defocus curve measurements through changes in higher-order aberrations, [37, 109] coupled with changes in exposure of the lens' optics, which may impact on the VA achieved. [36, 110] To overcome this limitation, it may be advantageous to measure defocus curves under different lighting conditions and with different letter contrasts to fully appreciate visual performance under different viewing conditions. However, performing such a comprehensive battery of tests can prove to be time-consuming and both visually and physically demanding for the subject. Other important considerations include correcting the VA results to account for the magnifying effect of the test lens' power and back vertex distance. [89, 100]

Defocus curves have been frequently used to demonstrate improvements in the focusing range provided by presbyopic IOLs compared to monofocal IOLs, [50, 97-99, 111-114] and to differentiate between different presbyopia-correcting technologies. [106, 115] However, the evaluation of the amplitude of accommodation from defocus curves differs substantially between even carefully conducted studies, depending on the criteria used to define 'the range of clear vision'. [100] The direct comparison analysis method compares the VA achieved at each level of defocus, but is susceptible to type-1 errors, unless repeated-measures ANOVA or a Bonferroni correction is used.

Depth-of-focus metrics provide a general overview of the anticipated performance of an IOL. This is defined as the dioptric range over which subjects can sustain an absolute or relative level of VA. However, there is no general consensus for the correct threshold level of VA, and often the criteria used are not stated, preventing comparisons between studies. [100] A 'relative' criterion determines the cut-off point relative to the best-achieved VA. To date, relative acuity criteria have not been used in multifocal IOL studies, but have been used for assessment of accommodating IOLs. [113] A criterion of a +0.04 logMAR reduction in VA from the best-corrected distance acuity (to account for the variability of measurements made using a logMAR chart, which is relatively unaffected by age), [116] has been shown to give the most reliable results. [100] Alternatively, with 'absolute' acuity criteria, the limits of VA are independent of the best-corrected VA. A limit of +0.30 logMAR is the most common criterion used in multifocal IOL studies and matches the level of acuity defined as the driving standard across Europe. [117]

The two focal points created by the simultaneous bifocal and multifocal IOL designs result in a distinctive profile with two or more peaks of optimum acuity, one at distance and the other at the blur level corresponding to the near addition powers. [92] Thus, defocus curves demonstrate the magnitude of the near addition powers (i.e. the separation in dioptres between the distance and near/intermediate peaks), as well as the quality of vision at distance, near and intermediate distances. [118] Whilst a reduction in acuity of +0.04 logMAR has been shown to be most appropriate for pre-presbyopes and accommodative restoration procedures, the defocus curve of a simultaneous vision bifocal or multifocal IOL can pass through the depth-of-focus criterion several times. Therefore, a new area metric has been developed and validated, [119] based on the area between a +0.30 logMAR absolute cut-off (or range-of-focus) and the defocus curve calculated for the upper and lower limits of distance (-0.50 and +0.50 D), intermediate (-2.00 and -0.50 D) and near vision (-4.00 and -2.00 D); Figure 2. This introduces a method of standardisation that will allow a comparison of different presbyopia-correcting strategies.

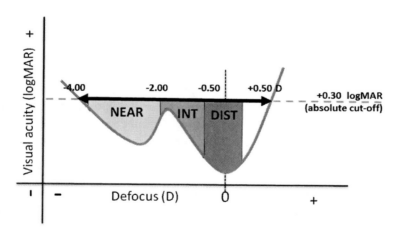

Figure 2. A schematic example of a 'typical' defocus curve from a presbyopia-correcting IOL demonstrating the absolute *'range-of-focus'* and three *'area-of-focus'* defocus curve metrics. The cut-off value of +0.30 logMAR is depicted by the horizontal dashed line. The black arrow depicts the *'range-of-focus'* metric using this 'absolute' acuity criterion. The left-hand zone under the curve represents the 'near' area metric (between 25 and 50 cm); the central zone under the curve represents the 'intermediate' (INT) area metric (between 50 cm and 2 m), and the right-hand zone under the curve represents the 'distance' (DIST) area metric.

5.1.2. Near Point Measurement (RAF Rule)

The RAF rule has long been used to measure accommodation for patients implanted with accommodating IOLs. [99, 113, 120] However, this method is known to over-estimate the true amplitude of the response, due to the increasing target visual angle as it is brought closer towards the eyes and changes in external illuminance. [121, 122]

5.2. Objective Measurement of Accommodation

Although subjective tests are useful to quantify patient satisfaction, these methods cannot discriminate between true accommodation and pseudoaccommodation due to other factors such as a reduction in pupil size. Objective methods to assess dynamic accommodation include autorefraction, retinoscopy, aberrometry and imaging any movement of the implanted IOL optics.

5.2.1. Retinoscopy

This method allows the operator to visualise changes in dioptric power as the patient looks at targets positioned over a range of different distances. [98, 99, 120, 123] However, this manual procedure relies on the observer's subjective interpretation of the light-reflex which may lead to a poor reproducibility of results between different practitioners. [124]

5.2.2. Autorefraction

Previous reports have measured changes in refractive power for patients implanted with accommodating IOLs using open-field autorefractors, [125] with the patient viewing static [113, 126-129] or dynamic accommodative targets. [126] However, pupillary constriction, either through senile miosis or through attempted accommodation, causes a hindrance for autorefractors. Minimum pupil diameters for autorefractor devices typically range between 2.3 mm (Shin-Nippon NVision-K5001/Grand Seiko WR-5100K and Grand Seiko Auto Ref/Keratometer WAM 5500) and 2.9 mm (Shin-Nippon SRW-5000/Grand Seiko WV-500). [125] Difficulties in capturing data through small pupils, coupled with bright Purkinje image reflections off the anterior IOL surface, or even potential posterior capsular opacification, may limit the usefulness of autorefractors in evaluating accommodation changes. [130] Nonetheless, Wolffsohn et al. [128] have demonstrated that the Shin-Nippon NVision-K5001/Grand Seiko WR-5100K device provides repeatable measurements of accommodation, comparable to subjective refraction data. In comparing objective and subjective measurements, other reports have shown that subjective methods tend to overestimate accommodation compared to autorefraction data. [99, 131, 132] This was to be expected, as subjective measurements include the added benefit of an increased depth-of-field due to pupillary miosis.

The PowerRefractor device (PlusOptix, Nuremberg, Germany) has been used to evaluate accommodating IOLs. [98, 99, 126] This instrument can provide continuous objective measures of refraction and pupil size for both eyes simultaneously, using eccentric photorefraction, with the camera positioned at a distance of 1 m from the patient. [133] Refractive results are calculated based on the light intensity distribution within the pupil, which cannot be precisely predicted between subjects, therefore individual calibration needs to be performed for accurate results. [133] Similar to autorefractors, evaluations of accommodation made with the PowerRefractor are achieved by measuring refraction whilst the patient fixates on distance and near targets. [99]

5.2.3. Change in IOL Optic Axial Position or Shape

An evaluation of any change in anterior chamber depth (ACD) or IOL optic surface shape upon ciliary body contraction can also be used as an indicator of IOL accommodative ability. Various methods of biometric assessment have been employed including anterior segment optical coherence tomography (AS-OCT), [113, 129, 134] partial coherence interferometry, [135] ultrasound biomicroscopy, [136, 137] and Scheimpflug imaging (Zeiss IOL master; Carl Zeiss Meditec, Jena, Germany). [99, 120] Whilst these methods can accurately image an axial shift in the IOL optic, or a change of crystalline lens surface curvature, they do not provide a direct measurement of a change in the refractive power of the eye.

Some investigations have used 2% Pilocarpine eye-drops to stimulate the ciliary body to induce accommodation to allow accommodating IOL optic axial movement analysis. [99, 135, 136] An advantage of pharmacological, rather than stimulus-driven accommodation, is that it does not require patient compliance to focus on a near target. [135] However, the subsequent powerful ciliary body contraction is coupled with marked pupillary constriction, [138] which hinders the measurement of objective refraction changes. [139] Furthermore, pharmacological stimulation of accommodation is not representative of the normal physiologic accommodative response, [135, 140] but may demonstrate the maximum potential accommodative ability of an accommodative IOL rather than its habitual performance.

5.2.4. Aberrometry

Similar to autorefractors, aberrometers can be used to measure objective changes in accommodation. An objective refraction is obtained by converting the second-order Zernike terms into the corresponding defocus and astigmatic components. [39] These devices have the advantage that as well as assessing central optical changes, the wavefront aberrations over the whole pupil aperture can also be quantified. Unfortunately, few are open-field, making them susceptible to instrument myopia, [141] but some use an internal Badal optical system to blur the subject to infinity. [142]

Most aberrometers operate over a narrow wavelength range (typically around 780-820 nm) and, therefore, require a correction to adjust measurements to equate to a wavelength of approximately 550 nm (the peak of the human spectral sensitivity curve). [143] Each set of captured wavefront errors are specific to a given pupil size only. Therefore, to facilitate comparisons between different subjects, measurements must be rescaled to the smallest pupil size common to all subjects. Alternatively, measurements can be recalculated into dioptric equivalents terms; however, this method requires separate data calculations. [144] As with autorefraction data, subjective tests tend to overestimate measurements of amplitude of accommodation compared to objective aberrometry. [132, 145, 146]

In summary, the evaluation of accommodating IOLs should include objective measures of both biometric and refractive changes, avoiding the instillation of Pilocarpine, to verify the existence of true pseudophakic accommodation. [130, 139] Subjective measures are also essential in regard to clinical outcomes, but these should not be interpreted in isolation. Most studies of accommodating IOLs have reported only subjective findings or have used Pilocarpine drops to stimulate accommodation to record objective changes in ACD. Currently, only a few studies have measured objective changes in refraction and IOL position. [113, 129] In general, there is a requirement for objective accommodation measurement techniques to be standardised to allow widespread use and acceptance. [130, 147, 148]

6. Estimating Optical Quality

Higher-order aberration measurements have been frequently used to explore the optical quality of eyes implanted IOLs. [66, 149, 150] The most commonly used optical quality metric is higher-order root-mean-square (RMS) wavefront error, however, RMS error does not provide any information regarding the magnitude or sign of individual aberration coefficient terms. [151] Modulation transfer function (MTF) has been used to explore the effectiveness of correcting spherical aberration using aspheric IOL designs, [149, 150, 152-156] but it cannot account for important factors affecting visual performance such as neural processing and patient adaptation. Arguably, the Strehl ratio metric may provide more useful information, as it evaluates performance compared to an ideal, diffraction-limited system. [150, 153, 154] Nonetheless, such image quality metrics are also specific to only one pupil size. In this regard, it can be useful to dilate the subject's pupils before capturing wavefront aberrations, as this facilitates analysis over a range of pupil sizes. However, it may be argued that pupillary dilation creates a 'non-habitual' scenario, influencing the phakic subject's ability to drive and/or read after measurements, particularly if a cycloplegic drug is used to achieve mydriasis. Carkeet et al. [157] reported small, yet significant, differences between higher-order aberration measurements following pupil dilation with cycloplegic and non-cycloplegic eye drops and changes in the location of the pupil centre occur following pupil dilation. [158] Other authors have reported that retinal image plane metrics correlate better with visual performance; [159, 160] however, these require separate data computation using additional software (GetMetrics; University of Houston, College of Optometry).

The Optical Quality Analysis System, or OQAS device, (VisioMetrics, Terrassa, Spain) uses the double-pass technique to evaluate intraocular light scatter and retinal image quality. Unlike the Hartmann-Shack technique, the OQAS device directly captures an image of the point source projected onto the retina, therefore, the captured images represent the point-spread function (PSF). Generation of a global PSF with the Hartmann-Shack technique requires computational reconstruction of the wave aberration leaving the eye, through complex evaluations of each individual spot image location captured at the wavefront sensor's charge-coupled device (CCD) camera. Spot imaging errors (e.g. spot image 'crossover') at the sensor may cause inaccuracies resulting in an under- or overestimation of optical quality. [161] Additionally, analysis of the captured spot image locations does not fully describe important optical phenomena such as scatter.

The main visual metrics outputted by the OQAS device include,

- Modulation transfer function (MTF) cut-off value – the highest spatial frequency (in cycles per degree) at which the eye can image an object on the retina with a contrast of 1 %
- Objective scattering index (OSI) – an objective measure of intraocular scatter, comparing the amount of light falling outside the double-pass retinal intensity PSF and the amount of light at the centre of the PSF. Generally, the higher the OSI, the larger the magnitude of scatter [162]
- Two-dimensional (2-D) Strehl ratio – the ratio of the PSF's central maximum achieved by the measured (aberrated) eye compared to the theoretical maximum achieved by an 'ideal', aberration-free optical system
- PSF width – the width of the PSF (in minutes of arc) can be measured along various points of the function, e.g. the 'half-height' metric is the width of the PSF at 50 % of the maximal height.

The repeatability of the these metrics have been found to be good by some researchers, [163, 164] but poorer by others, [165] perhaps due to variations in the tear film [166-168] or in eyes with larger magnitudes of scatter, such as eyes with dense cataracts [162] and post-LASIK eyes. [164] Furthermore, the OQAS device uses near infrared light (approximately 780 nm), although this provides comfortable fixational viewing conditions during measurements, infrared light penetrates deeper into the retinal tissues causing larger magnitudes of scatter. [169]

The OQAS instrument's entrance pupil is typically fixed at a diameter of approximately 2 mm, whereas the exit pupil diameter is adjustable (between 2 and 7 mm) facilitating the derivation and interpretation of non-rotationally-symmetric aberrations. [170-172] The PSF is classically obtained through phase-retrieval algorithms which combine two double-pass retinal images. [173] The first retinal image is captured using equivalent-sized entrance and exit pupil diameters (i.e. 2 mm) and the second captured when the entrance pupil is smaller in diameter than the exit pupil, resulting in a lower resolution PSF than when the pupil sizes were equivalent. This computational process can cause inaccuracies when evaluating optical quality with diffractive multifocal IOLs, especially as most lens designs feature their first diffractive step within the central 2 mm. Additionally, the double-pass technique assumes that the incident light of the first pass is minimally affected by the eyes' optics, which is not the case for those implanted with diffractive IOLs. [169]

When comparing MTFs measured with the double-pass method vs. the Hartmann-Shack technique (both with a wavelength of 780 nm), similar results were found in young, visually-normal subjects with low magnitudes of intraocular scatter, but the Hartmann-Shack method typically over-estimated retinal image quality in older patients with early lenticular opacities, post-LASIK patients and post-IOL implantation patients. [174] Moreover, the MTFs obtained with the double-pass method showed better correlation with VA compared to the MTFs measured using the Hartmann-Shack technique. A similar trend was also reported when comparing optical quality measured with the double-pass method and the laser ray-tracing (LRT) technique, both using a wavelength of 532 nm. [175]

7. IOL Rotation, Tilt and Decentration

Accurate positioning and alignment of an IOL with respect to the visual axis is critical to ensure optimal correction of refractive error and spherical aberration. Unwanted IOL tilt and decentration of multifocal, aspheric or toric IOLs has a significantly higher impact on visual function compared to spherical, monofocal IOLs. [176, 177] Possible sources of post-implantation positional errors include:

- Friction between the IOL haptics and the capsular bag, dependant on the capsule and IOL size
- Compression of the IOL haptics due to capsular bag shrinkage
- Instability of the anterior chamber due to variations in post-operative IOP and ocular trauma
- Aspects of the IOL design, e.g. plate or loop style haptics, IOL and/or haptic materials and the overall haptic diameter

Other factors affecting IOL positional stability include the capsular bag diameter, [178, 179] capsulorhexis size, anterior and posterior capsule apposition, [180] IOL design [181, 182] and IOL material. [183, 184] In addition, Shah et al. [185] found that eyes with longer axial lengths had higher magnitudes of toric IOL rotation than eyes with shorter axial lengths. This agrees with Vass et al.'s [179] previous study, which showed a relationship between axial length and capsular bag diameter.

7.1. Rotation

Previous studies evaluating the rotational stability of toric IOLs have used a slit-lamp eye-piece (with an integrated axis indicator graticule) [186, 187] or a slit-beam protractor. [181, 188, 189] Although useful, these slit-lamp-based techniques are dependent on the patient maintaining a stable, erect head position at each assessment visit, and are usually limited to estimating axis rotations to the nearest 5 degrees only.

Other studies have used digital slit-lamp images to investigate toric axis stability; [182, 190-192] however, no compensation for axis alterations, due to either head tilt and/or ocular rotation, were made. Recent techniques have employed image-analysis of digital photographs, using customised software, in an attempt to eliminate these errors. [185, 193-195] Such imaging techniques compare the position of the toric axis alignment markers with easily distinguishable ocular landmarks, such as episcleral blood vessels or iris features, on opposite sides of the pupil margins, to normalise for any eye rotation. Furthermore, image-overlaying analysis software can also be used to determine the magnitude of any potential IOL decentration by comparing the centre of the outlined IOL optic edge, the pupil margin and the limbal margin. [185, 193, 194]

7.2. Tilt and Decentration

Several reports have described the use of Scheimpflug imaging to evaluate IOL tilt and centration within the capsular bag using the EAS-1000 device (Nidek Inc., Gamagori, Japan) [196-200] and the Oculus Pentacam (Oculus, Wetzlar, Germany). [176, 201-203] Both instruments are designed so that the image and object planes are tilted with respect to each other to intersect at a point, allowing the entire object to be sharply focussed. [204] As light passes through the eye and through the tilt of the Scheimpflug camera, the unprocessed Scheimpflug image will be distorted due to refraction through the corneal surfaces. [87, 205, 206] Therefore, a correction factor must be applied before evaluating IOLs images; however, it is difficult to accurately account for the effects of hydration and variations in refractive index within such ocular tissues. [202, 207]

The tilt angle of the IOL optical axis relative to the eye's visual axis is estimated using specialised software which evaluates various points along both the anterior corneal and anterior IOL surfaces of corrected Scheimpflug images. Using this imaging technique, previous studies have demonstrated that IOL tilting induces unwanted 3rd-order coma. [177, 208] Nonetheless, the Scheimpflug imaging method to estimate IOL tilt and rotation does not include compensations for any potential tilting of the head or ocular cyclotorsion during image capture. In this regard, the observer has to ensure that the patient's head is kept as erect and vertically aligned as is possible for each measurement/visit. [209]

Another technique used to assess IOL tilt and decentration includes evaluating Purkinje image reflections (P) off the ocular refracting surfaces. [201, 210-213] The radius of curvature of the different ocular components (acting as mirrors) can be estimated from the relative position of the reflected images of the light source. The first (P1: air-tear film-cornea) and second (P2: cornea-aqueous) Purkinje images are typically similar in size and usually overlap, due to the close proximity of the corneal surfaces. The aqueous-lens reflection (P3) is usually the largest in size (approximately twice P1) and finally the lens-vitreous reflection (P4) is usually slightly smaller than P1; however, it is inverted with respect to the other images. [201]

Purkinje image misalignment is due to a combination of global eye rotation, crystalline lens decentration and tilting of the crystalline lens. [211] Purkinje imaging allows evaluation of lens tilt and decentration without the need for image distortion corrections; however, multiple double LEDs of differing separation are required to prevent over-estimations of the posterior lens radius of curvature. [201, 213] Tabernero et al. [211] designed a custom-built Purkinjemeter using a semi-circular array of 9 infrared LEDs to illuminate the eye co-aligned with a telecentric camera objective lens and a CCD camera. The use of a semi-circular light source offers several advantages over a point source; e.g. the generated reflections show a non-symmetric geometry, allowing simple identification of each Purkinje image even when partially reduced in intensity by the pupil. Furthermore, multiple LEDs allow estimates of the radii of curvature as a function of radial distance and therefore, estimates of asphericity. In order to determine IOL centration, customised image-processing software is typically used to determine the location of each Purkinje image with respect to the centre of the entrance pupil (fitted to an ellipse).

In comparing Scheimpflug and Purkinje imaging in the same population, Rosales et al. [201] reported higher variability with the Purkinje image technique. Purkinje imaging can evaluate both lens surfaces, whereas Scheimpflug imaging is hindered by the iris, particularly with increased accommodation. Nonetheless, Scheimpflug imaging provides much more complete information on the biometry of the anterior chamber and lens geometry, beyond radius of curvature. On the other hand, the Purkinje imaging method is easier to set-up and to incorporate into existing optical systems incurring relatively low costs.

8. Stereopsis

In addition to optical quality and visual performance, accurate co-ordination of the two eyes is crucial for near vision manipulation tasks. Of the various near vision stereoacuity instruments available, the Wirt rings of the Titmus contour test (Stereo Optical Co. Inc.; Chicago, IL, US) appear to have been most frequently used to assess stereopsis in patients bilaterally-implanted with multifocal IOLs, [214-218] or monofocal IOLs. [216, 219] In contrast, Random Dot tests (e.g. the Lang tests I and II; Oculus, Wetzlar, Germany) have been used for evaluating monofocal and multifocal IOLs implanted unilaterally. [220, 221] Although useful in adult patients, stereoacuity measurements are invaluable in paediatric patients implanted with IOLs.

9. Evaluation of Scatter (Haloes and Glare)

9.1. Forward Light Scatter (FLS) and Intraocular Straylight

Inhomogeneities of the optical media, e.g. within the crystalline lens, cause alterations in the trajectory of light rays passing through the eye. Scattered light deviated by less than 90 degrees is known as forward light scatter (FLS), which results in a veiling luminance becoming superimposed upon the retinal image, leading to a reduction in retinal image contrast and possible disability glare. [222] When assessing the optical quality of multifocal IOLs, it is important to differentiate between scatter and glare. Scatter is an optical phenomenon dependent on the intensity and wavelength of the incident light, and the optical and geometrical properties of the scattering structure (e.g. refractive index, spatial distribution, size and shape). On the other hand, glare refers to a subjective perception, where there is excessive contrast loss or an inappropriate distribution of light disturbing the ability to distinguish detail. For normal eyes, FLS represents around 1 to 2 % of the incident light falling outside the 'ideal' position on the retina. [222] Scattering is usually attributed to the cornea, crystalline lens and fundus, [223] although the iris and the sclera may also contribute towards a small proportion of FLS, depending on the patient's ethnicity. [224]

Objective measurements of FLS can be made using the van den Berg Straylight meter and the Oculus C-Quant (Oculus; Wetzlar, Germany) device. The C-Quant device is based on the van den Berg Straylight meter; however, unlike its predecessor, which uses the 'direct comparison' method, the C-Quant device uses the faster and more user-friendly forced-choice, 'compensation comparison' method. [225, 226] Coppens et al. [225] have demonstrated that the 'compensation comparison' method improves measurement repeatability and reliability. In support of this, other reports have suggested that the C-Quant device may be a suitable device for use in large scale clinical studies. [226, 227]

Theoretical predictions based on model eyes have suggested that diffractive multifocal IOLs induce more FLS than monofocal IOLs, [228] due to loss of light at higher diffractive orders. [229] In support of this, a number of studies have demonstrated that a small proportion of patients implanted with multifocal IOLs complain of photic phenomena, such as haloes and glare. [106, 230-233] However, increases in FLS (C-Quant) induced by multifocal IOLs do not appear to correlate with subjectively-reported glare symptoms, [230, 232, 233] perhaps indicating insensitivity of the C-Quant technique.

9.2. Halometry

When viewing a distant target, haloes are formed as the out-of-focus image from the near portion of a multifocal IOL typically shows a larger diameter than the sharper image focussed at the retina by the distance portion of the lens. Factors governing the size of the halo include the patient's pupil diameter, the multifocal IOL's near addition power, the distance power and the patient's corneal power. [234] Halometry involves quantifying the size of the halo created by a bright central light along multiple meridians. The Glare & Halo computer program (Tomey; Nagoya, Japan) involves marking of the edge of the perceived halo, generating an area metric, which has been used to compare the size of haloes experienced by patients implanted with multifocal versus monofocal IOLs. [234, 235] Pieh et al.'s [234] results showed that the Glare & Halo program demonstrated a high level of repeatability. However, the edge of a halo is often poorly defined, therefore complicating the subject's identification task. Also, small head or eye (fixational) movements may also result in a shift in the spatial location of the perceived halo. Furthermore, the computational algorithm used to calculate the halo's area is likely to assume that the halo has a circular ring shape; however, this assumption breaks down for eyes implanted with non-rotationally symmetric IOLs. An alternative approach, with high intra-session repeatability, has been introduced by Buckhurst et al. [236] Here a series of randomised letter targets are moved from a central LED towards the periphery along 8 different radial axes (in 45-degree steps), with the patient identifying when they are first seen. The target letters can be displayed at different sizes and levels of contrast. Buckhurst et al. [236] found that for patients implanted with non-rotationally symmetric multifocal IOLs, the perceived photic scotomas complemented the orientation of the IOL's reading segment, whereas fully-diffractive IOLs induced uniform photic scotomas.

10. Quality of Life (QOL) Questionnaires

Several questionnaires have been designed to investigate quality-of-life (QOL) in patients with cataract. Although the majority of these instruments have not been specifically developed for pseudophakic patients, they have been used in a variety of IOL-implanted populations in an attempt to standardise patient reported visual outcomes, such as post-operative spectacle dependence, driving ability and the ability to perform various social activities. [237, 238] Table 2 summarises these instruments, their target audience, which traits they explore and their validation (where appropriate).

10.1. The Cataract Type Specification

This instrument was first modified and validated by Javitt et al. [239] in a comparative study of patients implanted bilaterally with multifocal IOLs versus patients implanted bilaterally with monofocal IOLs. Javitt et al. [240] found that the instrument's internal consistency did not vary by method of administration (by self-administration at the site of care (pre-operative) and by mail (post-operative)), race or gender, for patients undergoing first eye cataract surgery. The instrument investigates visual functioning across 5 scales: distance vision, near vision, daytime driving, night driving and glare-related symptoms. Gothwal et al.'s [241] study performed Rasch analysis [242] on data collected from patients awaiting cataract surgery. Gothwal et al.'s [241] results showed that only 2 of the 5 scales were valid and a revised version was developed consisting of 11 items.

10.2. The Near Activity Visual Questionnaire (NAVQ)

Following a pilot study by Gupta et al., [243] Buckhurst and co-workers [244] modified and validated a questionnaire designed to assess near visual function for patients implanted with presbyopic corrections, from spectacles and contact lenses, to multifocal IOLs. Following Rasch analysis, the original number of items was reduced from 19 to 10 (and the scale of responses from 6 to 4). The author's results demonstrated that the instrument was internally consistent, valid and reliable in their subject population. Buckhurst et al. [244] also reported moderate correlations of NAVQ scores with both near VA and CPS scores, further highlighting the need for such questionnaires to contribute to the evaluation of the subjective perception of successful presbyopia correction.

10.3. The Quality of Vision (QoV) Questionnaire

This instrument was developed and evaluated by McAlinden et al. [245] The QoV questionnaire is a linear-scaled, 30-item instrument providing a QoV score in terms of symptom frequency, severity, and how bothersome the symptom is. The instrument appears to be suitable for measuring QoV in patients with all types of laser refractive correction, intraocular refractive surgery and eye diseases that cause QoV problems.

10.4. The Visual Function Index-14 (VF-14) QOL Questionnaire

Originally designed by Steinberg et al., [246] this questionnaire has been validated to assess functional impairment in cataract patients before and after monofocal IOL implantation. [247] Other authors have used this instrument to evaluate visual outcomes in comparative studies of patients implanted with monofocal versus multifocal IOLs. [248, 249] Uusitalo et al. [250] proposed the exclusion of 7 items from the original questionnaire; this modified version, the VF-7 survey, has since been used to compare surgical outcomes for patients implanted with multifocal IOLs versus patients fitted with conventional monofocal IOLs. [251] Recently, Gothwal et al. [252] validated this 7-item questionnaire using Rasch analysis to assess its psychometric properties, and led to the development of an improved 8-item instrument.

10.5. The Catquest-9SF Instrument

The Catquest-9SF test was initially developed and validated by Lundstrom et al. [253] and consisted of 17 items across 4 subscales. The instrument has previously been used to measure changes in patient-reported visual function 6 months after cataract surgery compared to before surgery. [254] Furthermore, Lundstrom and Pesudovs [255] validated the psychometric properties of the instrument using data collected from 10,486 completed questionnaires (before and after cataract surgery) and found improved performance with a revised 9-item version, consisting of 7 functioning items and 2 global items.

10.6. Adapted National Eye Institute Visual Function Questionnaire-25 (NEI-VFQ-25)

Originally developed by Mangione et al., [256] the NEI-VFQ comprised 51 items to evaluate a broad spectrum of eye diseases. In a later study, Mangione et al. [257] compared a simpler, 25-item version of the test (the NEI-VFQ-25) against the original survey, and found comparable validity between instruments. Kohnen et al. [258] constructed a newer questionnaire by adapting sections from the near activities, distance activities and driving subscales of the original NEI-VFQ-25 test. Although Kohnen et al.'s [258] instrument has not yet been validated, it has been used to evaluate visual outcomes for patients implanted with multifocal IOLs. [106, 259]

10.7. The Visual Symptoms and Quality of Life (VSQ) Questionnaire

This instrument is available as a 14-item short form and a more detailed 26-item long form. The short form consists of 2 subscales for (1) symptoms and visual dysfunction, and (2) vision-specific QOL items. [260] Donovan et al.'s [260] validation study was performed on patients requiring 'second' eye cataract surgery randomised to either receive early (within six weeks) or routine surgery (7–12 months on a waiting list), with a follow-up visit approximately six months after surgery, to evaluate the effectiveness of second eye cataract surgery. The results showed that the internal consistency of both the visual symptoms/dysfunction and QOL items was high.

Aside from these validated instruments, the use of questionnaires specifically exploring the appearance and prevalence of photic phenomena, such as haloes and glare, appear to be growing in popularity for studies of multifocal IOLs. Several authors have implemented their own questionnaires; [230, 231, 234, 235, 261-264] however, some reports do not fully disclose what questions were asked, [89, 230] or how the results were graded. [234] Although other studies have revealed the questions asked and the grading systems applied to the answers, [231, 235, 261, 263, 264] their results have not been scientifically validated. Furthermore, the proposed responses may not always use a continuous interval level. When attempting to quantify such data, scoring from 'simple averaging' or 'summing of item responses' (e.g., 0, 1, 2, and 3 for responses such as 'not at all', 'a little', 'quite', and 'very', respectively) assumes that the quantitative differences between each response option is equal, and that each question has equivalent value. Both these assumptions may be invalid rendering the questionnaire scores as non-linear. [265]

The US Department of Health and Human Services Food and Drug Administration (FDA) has published specific guidelines relating to the development of patient-reported outcome measures. [266] This document provides specific guidance on recording evidence relating to the development history of questionnaires to ensure instruments adequately measure their intended outcomes. It also provides advice relating to design factors including the number of items, item discrimination, scoring methods, response ranges and translation or cultural adaptability of the questionnaire.

Table 2. A summary of questionnaires used in cataract and IOL-implanted patients

Questionnaire	Key references	Study population	Traits evaluated	Validation
Cataract TyPE Specification	Javitt et al., 2003 [240] Gothwal et al., 2009 [241]	Patients with cataract	Vision: daytime, night driving & glare	Rasch analysis
The Quality of Vision (QoV) Questionnaire	McAlinden et al., 2010 [245]	All types of refractive correction & eye diseases that cause QoV problems	Photic phenomena: Glare, haloes, starbursts, distortion, diplopia, focussing & depth perception	Rasch analysis
The Visual Function Index-14 (VF-14) QOL Questionnaire	Uusitalo et al., 1999 [250] Gothwal et al., 2010 [252]	Patients with cataract	Vision: for cooking, near tasks, mobility-related aspects & TV	Rasch analysis
The Catquest-9SF Instrument	Lundstrom et al., 1997 [253] Lundstrom and Pesudovs, 2009 [255]	Cataract patients pre- and post-op	Reading tasks, watching TV, recognising faces	Rasch analysis
Adapted National Eye Institute Visual Function Questionnaire-25 (NEI-VFQ-25)	Kohnen et al., 2009 [258]	Used for a broad spectrum of eye disease e.g. glaucoma, ARMD	Vision (including colour and peripheral vision), driving, vision-specific expectations, vision-specific sole functioning.	Not yet validated
The Visual Symptoms and Quality of life (VSQ) Questionnaire	Donovan et al., 2003 [260]	Patients with cataract and patients awaiting 2nd eye cataract surgery	Difficulties in completing tasks e.g. driving, pouring liquids etc. How vision effects the patient's feelings about their present life and the future	Internal consistency (Cronbach's alpha)
The Near Activity Visual Questionnaire	Buckhurst et al., 2012 [244] Gupta et al., 2007 [243]	Patients fitted with presbyopic corrections including spectacles, contact lenses and IOLs	Near vision tasks, spectacles dependency & glare	Rasch analysis

11. Analysing Posterior Capsular Opacification (PCO)

Posterior capsule opacification (PCO) is still the most common complication of modern cataract surgery. Although its incidence has decreased slightly, because of improved surgical technique and new IOL designs, the reported incidence is still substantial and varies greatly, from 18.4 to 38.4 % up to 5 years after surgery. [267] A variety of systems have been used to analyse PCO, however, no single system has been endorsed as the 'gold standard'. The oldest technique employed is based on clinical grading using slit-lamp biomicroscopy. Although extensively used, the subjective and qualitative nature of this technique is dependent on the experience of the examiner. Also, there is no universally-accepted subjective grading scale for PCO, with different authors suggesting the use of various grading categories. [268-270] Nonetheless, clinical grading has been shown to correlate well with some objective methods. [271] It is expected that image-analysis techniques, such as Scheimpflug and digital photographic imaging, will provide more reliable and accurate assessments of PCO.

11.1. Scheimpflug Imaging

Both Hayashi at al. [272] and Lasa et al. [273] have used the EAS-1000 device (Nidek, Gamagori, Japan) equipped with area densitometry software to objectively measure the intensity of light scattering (considered to be equal to the opacification density). However, this Scheimpflug device only allows opacification density values to be evaluated within the central 3.0 mm of the posterior capsule. [272] To date, only Hayashi et al. [272] have reported correlations between opacification density values and VA for patients with PCO. As this device can only evaluate slit sections, there is scope for missing areas of PCO if they do not lie within the analysed meridian. Therefore, the restricted number of axes analysed limits comprehensive PCO evaluation with the EAS-1000 device. Grewal and colleagues [274] have used the Oculus Pentacam, a rotating Scheimpflug camera, to evaluate PCO, as this instrument captures images along multiple meridians. Currently, however, no studies have used the Pentacam to monitor PCO progression. [275]

11.2. Digital Photography

As PCO essentially occurs along a single focal plane, retro-illuminated digital photographic images can be used for PCO analysis. Wang and Woung [276] used a computerised algorithm to analyse the brightness of different points of retro-illuminated, digital images from eyes with PCO. The software compared each graded point against a threshold transparency value, and calculated the percentage level of transparency over each point. However, several sources of error can occur with this method, including variations in background intensity, and also from factors such as differences in pupillary dilatation, fundus pigmentation and head position. [277] Clinical factors specific to pseudophakic eyes, such as IOL centration, tilt and differences in refractive indices between different IOL materials can also lead to artefacts of variable illumination. [278]

Freidman and co-workers [279] addressed some of the concerns raised regarding objective digital photography, by introducing a camera system based on cross-polarised illumination to supress reflections from the corneal surfaces. Uneven illumination was accounted for using specialised image processing software (IPLaboratory; Signal Analytics, Vienna, VA). Although useful, a Maltese cross-shaped artefact is often seen during image capture, thereby obstructing the examiners view.

Tetz and Nimsgern [280] developed the Evaluation of Posterior Capsular Opacification (EPCO) method, based on retro-illumination photographs captured using a standard slit lamp camera. The software allows morphological measurement of PCO through densitometry assessments across a 2-dimensional plane. The PCO density across different areas of the image is interactively outlined by the observer (using the software drawing tools) and scored on a scale from 0 to 4. The individual PCO score is calculated by multiplying the opacification grade by the fraction of the capsular area involved behind the IOL optic. Although this method is relatively inexpensive, it is not fully objective and relies on observer operation and interpretation. Therefore, it was perhaps not surprising that Findl et al. [271] reported significant correlations between EPCO scores and subjective grading scores made at the slit-lamp.

Barman et al. [281] have proposed another PCO image analysis technique, known as the POCO system, which classifies different areas of the image as either 'textured' or 'non-textured' using a semi-objective method after removal of the corneal Purkinje image reflections. The software algorithm applies image contrast enhancement filters to enhance the texture of any areas of opacity; images are then classified into areas of 'opacity' or 'transparency'. A major disadvantage of this method is that the areas of the image encompassing the Purkinje image reflections are completely excluded from the overall image analysis; this may be of significance if the areas of PCO are located centrally, as they may originally have been masked by the corneal reflections. In addition, this technique requires a specialised image capture and analysis system to capture the source images, which incurs additional expense. A similar device, known as the POCOman system, has been introduced by Bender et al. [282] However, this method also requires some subjective input as the observer is required to grade the texture of the image. Therefore, this aspect of the technique may introduce inaccuracies, as the skill of grading texture is likely to be dependent on the observer's clinical experience. [271]

To remove Purkinje reflections, Buehl et al. [283] have developed the Automated Quantification of After-Cataract (AQUA) imaging system. Here a series of retro-illumination images are captured whilst the patient fixates in slightly different directions, which essentially shifts the position of the Purkinje images. The resultant images are then fused together using sophisticated image analysis algorithms, based around 4 non-collinear points manually selected for image registration. [271] Although useful, this technique requires multiple images to be taken, increasing the time required for data collection.

Grewal and colleagues [274] used specialised medical imaging software (NIH ImageJ; National Institutes of Health, Bethesda, US) to analyse and compare Scheimpflug tomograms (Oculus Pentacam) versus data collected using the POCOman system, and found the results to be comparable.

In summary, objective methods of imaging PCO have evolved; however, a mixture of objective and subjective techniques is currently required to grade such opacities. Development of a fully objective grading system that captures IOL-capsular bag images along multiple meridians is desirable to monitor PCO progression and allow comparisons between studies.

Conclusion

As the technology used to design and manufacture IOLs improves, the need for long-term data relating to the performance of eyes implanted with IOLs also increases. A large proportion of IOL studies have assessed patients over time-spans ranging between 3 months [191] and 5 years, [284] with fewer studies extending beyond 2 years of follow-up. [285] Published reports beyond

10 years appear to be even sparser. [286] Development of a widely-accepted, comprehensive portfolio of assessments for evaluating IOL performance would be helpful in collecting long-term data from patients implanted with a variety of IOLs. Such long-term data would be useful for eyecare practitioners to better predict post-operative clinical outcomes and to manage patient expectations for those awaiting cataract surgery.

It is evident that several key measurements, including near VA, defocus curves and contrast sensitivity, require improved standardisation amongst the research community to allow better comparisons between studies. Aspects such as the target used; letter and lens sequence randomisation; the range of test lenses investigated and the number of spatial frequencies presented need to be considered. Recently, some researchers have attempted to combine a range of visual performance assessments into a single testing instrument, the Eyevispod system (PGB srl., Milano, Italy); to date, this device has only been used in one published study. [287]

Measurement of changes in accommodation (for eyes implanted with accommodative IOLs) should be conducted using both subjective and objective methods to determine whether increases in accommodation arise from actual changes in the IOL position, or due to changes in depth-of-field through pupillary constriction. It is also recommended that the evaluation of post-operative IOL centration and rotation uses a method which compares the IOL position to 'fixed' ocular landmarks, such as the episcleral blood vessels. Although a variety of QOL questionnaires have been used to assess the performance of IOLs, not all of these have yet been validated using methods such as Rasch analysis, [242] to ensure that each questionnaire item is measuring the desired characteristic.

In conclusion, this report reviews a variety of clinical assessment techniques typically used to evaluate the visual and optical performance of patients implanted with IOLs, highlighting their relative advantages and shortfalls. These findings should assist researchers in developing a comprehensive series of investigations designed to evaluate the performance of IOLs. Repeatable and reproducible *in-vivo* assessments of visual and optical performance are desirable to further develop IOL concepts and designs, in the hope of improving current post-operative visual satisfaction.

References

[1] Bailey IL & Lovie JE. New Design Principles for Visual Acuity Letter Charts. *Am J Optom Physiol Opt.* 1976;53:740-5.
[2] Regan D, Silver R & Murray TJ. Visual Acuity and Contrast Sensitivity in Multiple Sclerosis-Hidden Visual Loss: *An Auxiliary Diagnostic Test. Brain.* 1977;100:563-79.
[3] Ferris FL, Kassoff A, Bresnick GH & Bailey I. New Visual Acuity Charts for Clinical Research. *Am J Ophthalmol.* 1982;94:91-6.
[4] Brown B & Lovie-Kitchin JE. High and Low Contrast Acuity and Clinical Contrast Sensitivity Tested in a Normal Population. *Optom Vis Sci.* 1989;66:467-73.
[5] Regan D & Neima D. Low-Contrast Letter Charts in Early Diabetic Retinopathy, Ocular Hypertension, Glaucoma, and Parkinson's Disease. *Br J Ophthalmol.* 1984;68:885-9.
[6] International Organization for Standardization. *Ophthalmic Optics - Visual Acuity Testing - Standard Optotype and its Presentation.* ISO 8596. 1994.
[7] Hazel CA & Elliott DB. The Dependency of LogMAR Visual Acuity Measurements on Chart Design and Scoring Rule. *Optom Vis Sci.* 2002;79:788-92.
[8] Williams MA, Moutray TN & Jackson AJ. Uniformity of Visual Acuity Measures in Published Studies. *Invest Ophthalmol Vis Sci.* 2008;49:4321-7.
[9] Shah N, Laidlaw DA, Brown G & Robson C. Effect of Letter Separation on Computerised Visual Acuity Measurements: Comparison with the Gold Standard Early Treatment Diabetic Retinopathy Study (ETDRS) Chart. *Ophthalmic Physiol Opt.* 2010;30:200-3.
[10] Rosser DA, Murdoch IE, Fitzke FW & Laidlaw DA. Improving on ETDRS Acuities: Design and Results for a Computerised Thresholding Device. *Eye (Lond).* 2003;17:701-6.
[11] Sloan LL. New Test Charts for the Measurement of Visual Acuity at Far and near Distances. *Am J Ophthalmol.* 1959;48:807-13.
[12] Gupta N, Wolffsohn JS & Naroo SA. Comparison of near Visual Acuity and Reading Metrics in Presbyopia Correction. *J Cataract Refract Surg.* 2009;35:1401-9.
[13] Wolffsohn JS & Cochrane AL. The Practical near Acuity Chart (PNAC) and Prediction of Visual Ability at Near. *Ophthalmic Physiol Opt.* 2000;20:90-7.

[14] Bailey IL & Lovie JE. The Design and Use of a New near-Vision Chart. *Am J Optom Physiol Opt.* 1980;57:378-87.

[15] Sheedy JE, Subbaram MV, Zimmerman AB & Hayes JR. Text Legibility and the Letter Superiority Effect. *Hum Factors.* 2005;47:797-815.

[16] Liu L & Arditi A. How Crowding Affects Letter Confusion. *Optom Vis Sci.* 2001;78:50-5.

[17] Kniestedt C & Stamper RL. Visual Acuity and its Measurement. *Ophthalmol Clin North Am.* 2003;16:155-70.

[18] Kasper T, Buhren J & Kohnen T. Visual Performance of Aspherical and Spherical Intraocular Lenses: Intraindividual Comparison of Visual Acuity, Contrast Sensitivity, and Higher-Order Aberrations. *J Cataract Refract Surg.* 2006;32:2022-9.

[19] Ricci F, Scuderi G, Missiroli F, Regine F & Cerulli A. Low Contrast Visual Acuity in Pseudophakic Patients Implanted with an Anterior Surface Modified Prolate Intraocular Lens. *Acta Ophthalmol Scand.* 2004;82:718-22.

[20] Johansson B, Sundelin S, Wikberg-Matsson A, Unsbo P & Behndig A. Visual and Optical Performance of the Akreos Adapt Advanced Optics and Tecnis Z9000 Intraocular Lenses: Swedish Multicenter Study. *J Cataract Refract Surg.* 2007;33:1565-72.

[21] Thomson D. VA Testing in Optometric Practice. *Optom Today.* 2005;May:22-4.

[22] Laidlaw DA, Tailor V, Shah N, Atamian S & Harcourt C. Validation of a Computerised LogMAR Visual Acuity Measurement System (Complog): Comparison with ETDRS and the Electronic ETDRS Testing Algorithm in Adults and Amblyopic Children. *Br J Ophthalmol.* 2008;92:241-4.

[23] Thomson D. Near Vision Assessment in the 21st Century. *The Optician.* 2009;November:22-3.

[24] Beck RW, Moke PS, Turpin AH, et al. A Computerized Method of Visual Acuity Testing: Adaptation of the Early Treatment of Diabetic Retinopathy Study Testing Protocol. *Am J Ophthalmol.* 2003;135:194-205.

[25] Bland JM & Altman DG. Statistical Methods for Assessing Agreement between Two Methods of Clinical Measurement. *Int J Nursing Studies.* 2010;47:931-6.

[26] Cotter SA, Chu RH, Chandler DL, et al. Reliability of the Electronic Early Treatment Diabetic Retinopathy Study Testing Protocol in Children 7 to <13 Years Old. *Am J Ophthalmol.* 2003;136:655-61.
[27] Shah N, Laidlaw DA, Rashid S & Hysi P. Validation of Printed and Computerised Crowded Kay Picture LogMAR Tests against Gold Standard ETDRS Acuity Test Chart Measurements in Adult and Amblyopic Paediatric Subjects. *Eye (Lond).* 2012;26:593-600.
[28] Chen MT & Lin CC. Comparison of TFT-LCD and CRT on Visual Recognition and Subjective Preference. *Int J Indust Ergonomics.* 2004;34:167–74.
[29] Menozzi M, Lang F, Napflin U, Zeller C & Krueger H. CRT Versus LCD: Effects of Refrash Rate, Display Technology and Background Luminance in Visual Performance. *Displays.* 2001;22:79-85.
[30] Husain AM, Hayes S, Young M & Shah D. Visual Evoked Potentials with CRT and LCD Monitors: When Newer Is Not Better. *Neurology.* 2009;72:162-4.
[31] Thayaparan K, Crossland MD & Rubin GS. Clinical Assessment of Two New Contrast Sensitivity Charts. *Br J Ophthalmol.* 2007;91:749-52.
[32] Strasburger H, Wustenberg T & Jancke L. Calibrated LCD/TFT Stimulus Presentation for Visual Psychophysics in fMRI. *J Neurosci Methods.* 2002;121:103-10.
[33] Hollands JG, Parker HA, McFadden S & Boothby R. LCD Versus CRT Displays: A Comparison of Visual Search Performance for Colored Symbols. *Hum Factors.* 2002;44:210-21.
[34] Nagy BV, Gemesi S, Heller D, et al. Comparison of Pattern VEP Results Acquired Using CRT and TFT Stimulators in the Clinical Practice. *Doc Ophthalmol.* 2011;122:157-62.
[35] Lin YH, Chen CY, Lu SY & Lin YC. Visual Fatigue During VDT Work: Effects of Time-Based and Environment-Based Conditions. *Displays.* 2008;29:487-92.
[36] Oshika T, Okamoto C, Samejima T, Tokunaga T & Miyata K. Contrast Sensitivity Function and Ocular Higher-Order Wavefront Aberrations in Normal Human Eyes. *Ophthalmology.* 2006;113:1807-12.
[37] Liang J & Williams DR. Aberrations and Retinal Image Quality of the Normal Human Eye. *J Opt Soc Am A Opt Image Sci Vis.* 1997;14:2873-83.
[38] Thibos LN, Bradley A & Hong X. A Statistical Model of the Aberration Structure of Normal, Well-Corrected Eyes. *Ophthalmic Physiol Opt.* 2002;22:427-33.

[39] Thibos LN, Hong X, Bradley A & Cheng X. Statistical Variation of Aberration Structure and Image Quality in a Normal Population of Healthy Eyes. *J Opt Soc Am A Opt Image Sci Vis.* 2002;19:2329-48.

[40] Pesudovs K & Coster DJ. Assessment of Visual Function in Cataract Patients with a Mean Visual Acuity of 6/9. *Aust N Z J Ophthalmol.* 1996;24:5-9.

[41] Williamson TH, Strong NP, Sparrow J, Aggarwal RK & Harrad R. Contrast Sensitivity and Glare in Cataract Using the Pelli-Robson Chart. *Br J Ophthalmol.* 1992;76:719-22.

[42] Ravalico G, Baccara F & Rinaldi G. Contrast Sensitivity in Multifocal Intraocular Lenses. *J Cataract Refract Surg.* 1993;19:22-5.

[43] Campbell FW & Robson JG. Application of Fourier Analysis to the Visibility of Gratings. *J Physiol.* 1968;197:551-66.

[44] Packer M, Fine IH, Hoffman RS & Piers PA. Improved Functional Vision with a Modified Prolate Intraocular Lens. *J Cataract Refract Surg.* 2004;30:986-92.

[45] Bellucci R, Scialdone A, Buratto L, et al. Visual Acuity and Contrast Sensitivity Comparison between Tecnis and AcrySof SA60AT Intraocular Lenses: A Multicenter Randomized Study. *J Cataract Refract Surg.* 2005;31:712-7.

[46] Munoz G, Albarran-Diego C, Montes-Mico R, Rodriguez-Galietero A & Alio JL. Spherical Aberration and Contrast Sensitivity after Cataract Surgery with the Tecnis Z9000 Intraocular Lens. *J Cataract Refract Surg.* 2006;32:1320-7.

[47] Pandita D, Raj SM, Vasavada VA, Kazi NS & Vasavada AR. Contrast Sensitivity and Glare Disability after Implantation of AcrySof IQ Natural Aspherical Intraocular Lens: Prospective Randomized Masked Clinical Trial. *J Cataract Refract Surg.* 2007;33:603-10.

[48] Schmitz S, Dick HB, Krummenauer F, Schwenn O & Krist R. Contrast Sensitivity and Glare Disability by Halogen Light after Monofocal and Multifocal Lens Implantation. *Br J Ophthalmol.* 2000;84:1109-12.

[49] Ginsburg AP. A New Contrast Sensitivity Vision Test Chart. *Am J Optom Physiol Opt.* 1984;61:403-7.

[50] Steinert RF. Visual Outcomes with Multifocal Intraocular Lenses. *Curr Opin Ophthalmol.* 2000;11:12-21.

[51] Neumann AC, McCarty GR, Locke J & Cobb B. Glare Disability Devices for Cataractous Eyes: A Consumer's Guide. *J Cataract Refract Surg.* 1988;14:212-6.

[52] Prager TC, Urso RG, Holladay JT & Stewart RH. Glare Testing in Cataract Patients: Instrument Evaluation and Identification of Sources of Methodological Error. *J Cataract Refract Surg.* 1989;15:149-57.
[53] Reeves BC, Wood JM & Hill AR. Vistech Vcts 6500 Charts within- and between-Session Reliability. *Optom Vis Sci.* 1991;68:728-37.
[54] Pesudovs K, Hazel CA, Doran RM & Elliott DB. The Usefulness of Vistech and FACT Contrast Sensitivity Charts for Cataract and Refractive Surgery Outcomes Research. *Br J Ophthalmol.* 2004;88:11-6.
[55] Elliott DB & Bullimore MA. Assessing the Reliability, Discriminative Ability, and Validity of Disability Glare Tests. *Invest Ophthalmol Vis Sci.* 1993;34:108-19.
[56] Hong YT, Kim SW, Kim EK & Kim TI. Contrast Sensitivity Measurement with 2 Contrast Sensitivity Tests in Normal Eyes and Eyes with Cataract. *J Cataract Refract Surg.* 2010;36:547-52.
[57] McKee SP, Klein SA & Teller DY. Statistical Properties of Forced-Choice Psychometric Functions: Implications of Probit Analysis. *Percept Psychophys.* 1985;37:286-98.
[58] King-Smith PE, Grigsby SS, Vingrys AJ, Benes SC & Supowit A. Efficient and Unbiased Modifications of the Quest Threshold Method: Theory, Simulations, Experimental Evaluation and Practical Implementation. *Vision Res.* 1994;34:885-912.
[59] Kelly DH. Visual Contrast Sensitivity. *Optica Acta.* 1977;24:107-29.
[60] Montes-Mico R & Alio JL. Distance and Near Contrast Sensitivity Function after Multifocal Intraocular Lens Implantation. *J Cataract Refract Surg.* 2003;29:703-11.
[61] Kamlesh, Dadeya S & Kaushik S. Contrast Sensitivity and Depth of Focus with Aspheric Multifocal Versus Conventional Monofocal Intraocular Lens. *Can J Ophthalmol.* 2001;36:197-201.
[62] Montes-Mico R, Espana E, Bueno I, Charman WN & Menezo JL. Visual Performance with Multifocal Intraocular Lenses: Mesopic Contrast Sensitivity under Distance and near Conditions. *Ophthalmology.* 2004;111:85-96.
[63] Vingolo EM, Grenga P, Iacobelli L & Grenga R. Visual Acuity and Contrast Sensitivity: AcrySof ReSTOR Apodized Diffractive Versus AcrySof SA60AT Monofocal Intraocular Lenses. *J Cataract Refract Surg.* 2007;33:1244-7.
[64] Awwad ST, Warmerdam D, Bowman RW, et al. Contrast Sensitivity and Higher Order Aberrations in Eyes Implanted with AcrySof IQ SN60WF

and AcrySof SN60AT Intraocular Lenses. *J Refract Surg.* 2008;24:619-25.

[65] Caporossi A, Martone G, Casprini F & Rapisarda L. Prospective Randomized Study of Clinical Performance of 3 Aspheric and 2 Spherical Intraocular Lenses in 250 Eyes. *J Refract Surg.* 2007;23:639-48.

[66] Tzelikis PF, Akaishi L, Trindade FC & Boteon JE. Spherical Aberration and Contrast Sensitivity in Eyes Implanted with Aspheric and Spherical Intraocular Lenses: A Comparative Study. *Am J Ophthalmol.* 2008;145:827-33.

[67] Hutz WW, Eckhardt HB, Rohrig B & Grolmus R. Intermediate Vision and Reading Speed with Array, Tecnis, and ReSTOR Intraocular Lenses. *J Refract Surg.* 2008;24:251-6.

[68] Hutz WW, Eckhardt HB, Rohrig B & Grolmus R. Reading Ability with 3 Multifocal Intraocular Lens Models. *J Cataract Refract Surg.* 2006;32:2015-21.

[69] Brown D, Dougherty P, Gills JP, et al. Functional Reading Acuity and Performance: Comparison of 2 Accommodating Intraocular Lenses. *J Cataract Refract Surg.* 2009;35:1711-4.

[70] Ito M & Shimizu K. Reading Ability with Pseudophakic Monovision and with Refractive Multifocal Intraocular Lenses: Comparative Study. *J Cataract Refract Surg.* 2009;35:1501-4.

[71] Souza CE, Gerente VM, Chalita MR, et al. Visual Acuity, Contrast Sensitivity, Reading Speed, and Wavefront Analysis: Pseudophakic Eye with Multifocal IOL (ReSTOR) Versus Fellow Phakic Eye in Non-Presbyopic Patients. *J Refract Surg.* 2006;22:303-5.

[72] Souza CE, Muccioli C, Soriano ES, et al. Visual Performance of AcrySof ReSTOR Apodized Diffractive IOL: A Prospective Comparative Trial. *Am J Ophthalmol.* 2006;141:827-32.

[73] Radner W, Obermayer W, Richter-Mueksch S, et al. The Validity and Reliability of Short German Sentences for Measuring Reading Speed. *Graefes Arch Clin Exp Ophthalmol.* 2002;240:461-7.

[74] Subramanian A & Pardhan S. The Repeatability of MNRead Acuity Charts and Variability at Different Test Distances. *Optom Vis Sci.* 2006;83:572-6.

[75] Patel PJ, Chen FK, Da Cruz L, Rubin GS & Tufail A. Test-Retest Variability of Reading Performance Metrics Using MNRead in Patients with Age-Related Macular Degeneration. *Invest Ophthalmol Vis Sci.* 2011;52:3854-9.

[76] Virgili G, Pierrottet C, Parmeggiani F, et al. Reading Performance in Patients with Retinitis Pigmentosa: A Study Using the MNRead Charts. *Invest Ophthalmol Vis Sci.* 2004;45:3418-24.

[77] Finger RP, Charbel Issa P, Fimmers R, et al. Reading Performance Is Reduced by Parafoveal Scotomas in Patients with Macular Telangiectasia Type 2. *Invest Ophthalmol Vis Sci.* 2009;50:1366-70.

[78] Cheung SH, Kallie CS, Legge GE & Cheong AM. Nonlinear Mixed-Effects Modeling of MNRead Data. *Invest Ophthalmol Vis Sci.* 2008;49:828-35.

[79] Whittaker SG & Lovie-Kitchin J. Visual Requirements for Reading. *Optom Vis Sci.* 1993;70:54-65.

[80] Mansfield JS, Legge GE & Bane MC. A New Reading-Acuity Chart for Low and Normal Vision. *Opt Soc Am Techn Digest.* 1993;3:232-5.

[81] Pelli DG, Tillman KA, Freeman J, et al. Crowding and Eccentricity Determine Reading Rate. *J Vis.* 2007;7:20.1-36.

[82] Stifter E, Konig F, Lang T, et al. Reliability of a Standardized Reading Chart System: Variance Component Analysis, Test-Retest and Inter-Chart Reliability. *Graefes Arch Clin Exp Ophthalmol.* 2004;242:31-9.

[83] Hahn GA, Penka D, Gehrlich C, et al. New Standardised Texts for Assessing Reading Performance in Four European Languages. *Br J Ophthalmol.* 2006;90:480-4.

[84] Wolffsohn JS, Bhogal G & Shah S. Effect of Uncorrected Astigmatism on Vision. *J Cataract Refract Surg.* 2011;37:454-60.

[85] Duane A. Normal Values of the Accommodation at All Ages. *J Am Med Assoc.* 1912;LIX:1010-3.

[86] Koretz JF, Cook CA & Kaufman PL. Accommodation and Presbyopia in the Human Eye. Changes in the Anterior Segment and Crystalline Lens with Focus. *Invest Ophthalmol Vis Sci.* 1997;38:569-78.

[87] Dubbelman M, van der Heijde GL & Weeber HA. The Thickness of the Aging Human Lens Obtained from Corrected Scheimpflug Images. *Optom Vis Sci.* 2001;78:411-6.

[88] Dubbelman M, Van der Heijde GL, Weeber HA & Vrensen GF. Changes in the Internal Structure of the Human Crystalline Lens with Age and Accommodation. *Vision Res.* 2003;43:2363-75.

[89] Pieh S, Kellner C, Hanselmayer G, et al. Comparison of Visual Acuities at Different Distances and Defocus Curves. *J Cataract Refract Surg.* 2002;28:1964-7.

[90] Schmidinger G, Geitzenauer W, Hahsle B, et al. Depth of Focus in Eyes with Diffractive Bifocal and Refractive Multifocal Intraocular Lenses. *J Cataract Refract Surg.* 2006;32:1650-6.
[91] Hayashi K, Manabe S & Hayashi H. Visual Acuity from Far to Near and Contrast Sensitivity in Eyes with a Diffractive Multifocal Intraocular Lens with a Low Addition Power. *J Cataract Refract Surg.* 2009;35:2070-6.
[92] Maxwell WA, Cionni RJ, Lehmann RP & Modi SS. Functional Outcomes after Bilateral Implantation of Apodized Diffractive Aspheric Acrylic Intraocular Lenses with a +3.0 or +4.0 Diopter Addition Power: Randomized Multicenter Clinical Study. *J Cataract Refract Surg.* 2009;35:2054-61.
[93] Alio JL, Pinero DP, Plaza-Puche AB & Chan MJ. Visual Outcomes and Optical Performance of a Monofocal Intraocular Lens and a New-Generation Multifocal Intraocular Lens. *J Cataract Refract Surg.* 2011;37:241-50.
[94] Alio JL, Plaza-Puche AB, Javaloy J & Ayala MJ. Comparison of the Visual and Intraocular Optical Performance of a Refractive Multifocal IOL with Rotational Asymmetry and an Apodized Diffractive Multifocal IOL. *J Refract Surg.* 2012;28:100-5.
[95] Alio JL, Plaza-Puche AB, Javaloy J, et al. Comparison of a New Refractive Multifocal Intraocular Lens with an Inferior Segmental near Add and a Diffractive Multifocal Intraocular Lens. *Ophthalmology.* 2012;119:555-63.
[96] Post CT, Jr. Comparison of Depth of Focus and Low-Contrast Acuities for Monofocal Versus Multifocal Intraocular Lens Patients at 1 Year. *Ophthalmology.* 1992;99:1658-63; discussion 63-4.
[97] Steinert RF, Post CT, Jr., Brint SF, et al. A Prospective, Randomized, Double-Masked Comparison of a Zonal-Progressive Multifocal Intraocular Lens and a Monofocal Intraocular Lens. *Ophthalmology.* 1992;99:853-60; discussion 60-1.
[98] Langenbucher A, Huber S, Nguyen NX, et al. Measurement of Accommodation after Implantation of an Accommodating Posterior Chamber Intraocular Lens. *J Cataract Refract Surg.* 2003;29:677-85.
[99] Langenbucher A, Seitz B, Huber S, Nguyen NX & Kuchle M. Theoretical and Measured Pseudophakic Accommodation after Implantation of a New Accommodative Posterior Chamber Intraocular Lens. *Arch Ophthalmol.* 2003;121:1722-7.

[100] Gupta N, Wolffsohn JS & Naroo SA. Optimizing Measurement of Subjective Amplitude of Accommodation with Defocus Curves. *J Cataract Refract Surg.* 2008;34:1329-38.
[101] Trager MJ, Vagefi RM & McLeod SD. A Mathematical Model for Estimating Degree of Accommodation by Defocus Curves. *Invest Ophthalmol Vis Sci.* 2005;46:B691 (E-Abstract 717).
[102] Buckhurst PJ, Wolffsohn JS, Naroo SA, et al. Multifocal Intraocular Lens Differentiation Using Defocus Curves. *Invest Ophthalmol Vis Sci.* 2012;53:3920-6.
[103] Finkelman YM, Ng JQ & Barrett GD. Patient Satisfaction and Visual Function after Pseudophakic Monovision. *J Cataract Refract Surg.* 2009;35:998-1002.
[104] Ito M, Shimizu K, Amano R & Handa T. Assessment of Visual Performance in Pseudophakic Monovision. *J Cataract Refract Surg.* 2009;35:710-4.
[105] Richter-Mueksch S, Weghaupt H, Skorpik C, Velikay-Parel M & Radner W. Reading Performance with a Refractive Multifocal and a Diffractive Bifocal Intraocular Lens. *J Cataract Refract Surg.* 2002;28:1957-63.
[106] Santhiago MR, Wilson SE, Netto MV, et al. Visual Performance of an Apodized Diffractive Multifocal Intraocular Lens with +3.00-D Addition: 1-Year Follow-Up. *J Refract Surg.* 2011;27:899-906.
[107] Iida Y, Shimizu K & Ito M. Pseudophakic Monovision Using Monofocal and Multifocal Intraocular Lenses: Hybrid Monovision. *J Cataract Refract Surg.* 2011;37:2001-5.
[108] Gupta N, Naroo SA & Wolffsohn JS. Is Randomisation Necessary for Measuring Defocus Curves in Pre-Presbyopes? *Cont Lens Anterior Eye.* 2007;30:119-24.
[109] Wang Y, Zhao K, Jin Y, Niu Y & Zuo T. Changes of Higher Order Aberration with Various Pupil Sizes in the Myopic Eye. *J Refract Surg.* 2003;19:S270-4.
[110] Applegate RA, Marsack JD, Ramos R & Sarver EJ. Interaction between Aberrations to Improve or Reduce Visual Performance. *J Cataract Refract Surg.* 2003;29:1487-95.
[111] Steinert RF, Aker BL, Trentacost DJ, Smith PJ & Tarantino N. A Prospective Comparative Study of the AMO Array Zonal-Progressive Multifocal Silicone Intraocular Lens and a Monofocal Intraocular Lens. *Ophthalmology.* 1999;106:1243-55.

[112] Legeais JM, Werner L, Abenhaim A & Renard G. Pseudo-accommodation: Biocomfold Versus a Foldable Silicone Intraocular Lens. *J Cataract Refract Surg.* 1999;25:262-7.
[113] Cleary G, Spalton DJ & Marshall J. Pilot Study of New Focus-Shift Accommodating Intraocular Lens. *J Cataract Refract Surg.* 2010;36:762-70.
[114] Heatley CJ, Spalton DJ, Hancox J, Kumar A & Marshall J. Fellow Eye Comparison between the 1CU Accommodative Intraocular Lens and the AcrySof MA30 Monofocal Intraocular Lens. *Am J Ophthalmol.* 2005;140:207-13.
[115] Toto L, Falconio G, Vecchiarino L, et al. Visual Performance and Biocompatibility of 2 Multifocal Diffractive IOLs: Six-Month Comparative Study. *J Cataract Refract Surg.* 2007;33:1419-25.
[116] Raasch TW, Bailey IL & Bullimore MA. Repeatability of Visual Acuity Measurement. *Optom Vis Sci.* 1998;75:342-8.
[117] Coeckelbergh TR, Brouwer WH, Cornelissen FW, Van Wolffelaar P & Kooijman AC. The Effect of Visual Field Defects on Driving Performance: A Driving Simulator Study. *Arch Ophthalmol.* 2002;120:1509-16.
[118] Hansen TE, Corydon L, Krag S & Thim K. New Multifocal Intraocular Lens Design. *J Cataract Refract Surg.* 1990;16:38-41.
[119] Wolffsohn JS, Buckhurst PJ, Shah S, Naroo SA & Davies LN. Evaluation of Multifocal Intraocular Lens Defocus Curves. *Invest Ophthalmol Vis Sci.* 2011;52:(E-Abstract 4772).
[120] Kuchle M, Seitz B, Langenbucher A, et al. Comparison of 6-Month Results of Implantation of the 1CU Accommodative Intraocular Lens with Conventional Intraocular Lenses. *Ophthalmology.* 2004;111:318-24.
[121] Ostrin LA & Glasser A. Accommodation Measurements in a Prepresbyopic and Presbyopic Population. *J Cataract Refract Surg.* 2004;30:1435-44.
[122] Rosenfield M & Cohen AS. Repeatability of Clinical Measurements of the Amplitude of Accommodation. *Ophthalmic Physiol Opt.* 1996;16:247-9.
[123] Macsai MS, Padnick-Silver L & Fontes BM. Visual Outcomes after Accommodating Intraocular Lens Implantation. *J Cataract Refract Surg.* 2006;32:628-33.

[124] Rutstein RP, Fuhr PD & Swiatocha J. Comparing the Amplitude of Accommodation Determined Objectively and Subjectively. *Optom Vis Sci.* 1993;70:496-500.

[125] Sheppard AL, Bashir A, Wolffsohn JS & Davies LN. Accommodating Intraocular Lenses: A Review of Design Concepts, Usage and Assessment Methods. *Clin Exp Optom.* 2010;93:441-52.

[126] Wolffsohn JS, Hunt OA, Naroo S, et al. Objective Accommodative Amplitude and Dynamics with the 1CU Accommodative Intraocular Lens. *Invest Ophthalmol Vis Sci.* 2006;47:1230-5.

[127] Dogru M, Honda R, Omoto M, et al. Early Visual Results with the 1CU Accommodating Intraocular Lens. *J Cataract Refract Surg.* 2005;31:895-902.

[128] Wolffsohn JS, Davies LN, Naroo SA, et al. Evaluation of an Open-Field Autorefractor's Ability to Measure Refraction and Hence Potential to Assess Objective Accommodation in Pseudophakes. *Br J Ophthalmol.* 2011;95:498-501.

[129] Wolffsohn JS, Davies LN, Gupta N, et al. Mechanism of Action of the Tetraflex Accommodative Intraocular Lens. *J Refract Surg.* 2010;26:858-62.

[130] Dick HB. Accommodative Intraocular Lenses: Current Status. *Curr Opin Ophthalmol.* 2005;16:8-26.

[131] Wolffsohn JS, Naroo SA, Motwani NK, et al. Subjective and Objective Performance of the Lenstec KH-3500 "Accommodative" Intraocular Lens. *Br J Ophthalmol.* 2006;90:693-6.

[132] Win-Hall DM & Glasser A. Objective Accommodation Measurements in Pseudophakic Subjects Using an Autorefractor and an Aberrometer. *J Cataract Refract Surg.* 2009;35:282-90.

[133] Hunt OA, Wolffsohn JS & Gilmartin B. Evaluation of the Measurement of Refractive Error by the Powerrefractor: A Remote, Continuous and Binocular Measurement System of Oculomotor Function. *Br J Ophthalmol.* 2003;87:1504-8.

[134] Davies LN, Gibson GA, Sheppard AL & Wolffsohn JS. In Vivo Biometric Evaluation of Phakic and Pseudophakic Eyes During Accommodation with Optical Coherence Tomography. *Invest Ophthalmol Vis Sci.* 2008;49:(E-Abstract 3777).

[135] Kriechbaum K, Findl O, Koeppl C, Menapace R & Drexler W. Stimulus-Driven Versus Pilocarpine-Induced Biometric Changes in Pseudophakic Eyes. *Ophthalmology.* 2005;112:453-9.

[136] Alio JL, Ben-nun J, Rodriguez-Prats JL & Plaza AB. Visual and Accommodative Outcomes 1 Year after Implantation of an Accommodating Intraocular Lens Based on a New Concept. *J Cataract Refract Surg.* 2009;35:1671-8.
[137] Marchini G, Mora P, Pedrotti E, et al. Functional Assessment of Two Different Accommodative Intraocular Lenses Compared with a Monofocal Intraocular Lens. *Ophthalmology.* 2007;114:2038-43.
[138] Myers GA & Stark L. Topology of the Near Response Triad. *Ophthalmic Physiol Opt.* 1990;10:175-81.
[139] Glasser A. Restoration of Accommodation: Surgical Options for Correction of Presbyopia. *Clin Exp Optom.* 2008;91:279-95.
[140] Uthoff D, Holland D, Hepper D, et al. Laserinterferometric Measurements of Accommodative Changes in the Position of an Optic-Shift Intraocular Lens. *J Refract Surg.* 2009;25:416-20.
[141] Cervino A, Hosking SL, Rai GK, Naroo SA & Gilmartin B. Wavefront Analyzers Induce Instrument Myopia. *J Refract Surg.* 2006;22:795-803.
[142] Jinabhai A, Radhakrishnan H & O'Donnell C. Repeatability of Ocular Aberration Measurements in Patients with Keratoconus. *Ophthalmic Physiol Opt.* 2011;31:588-94.
[143] Charman WN. Wavefront Technology: Past, Present and Future. *Cont Lens Anterior Eye.* 2005;28:75-92.
[144] Radhakrishnan H, Jinabhai A & O'Donnell C. Dynamics of Ocular Aberrations in Keratoconus. *Clin Exp Optom.* 2010; 93 164-74
[145] Cleary G, Spalton DJ & Gala KB. A Randomized Intraindividual Comparison of the Accommodative Performance of the Bag-in-the-Lens Intraocular Lens in Presbyopic Eyes. *Am J Ophthalmol.* 2010;150:619-27e1.
[146] Hancox J, Spalton D, Heatley C, Jayaram H & Marshall J. Objective Measurement of Intraocular Lens Movement and Dioptric Change with a Focus Shift Accommodating Intraocular Lens. *J Cataract Refract Surg.* 2006;32:1098-103.
[147] Buznego C & Trattler WB. Presbyopia-Correcting Intraocular Lenses. *Curr Opin Ophthalmol.* 2009;20:13-8.
[148] Win-Hall DM & Glasser A. Objective Accommodation Measurements in Prepresbyopic Eyes Using an Autorefractor and an Aberrometer. *J Cataract Refract Surg.* 2008;34:774-84.
[149] Piers PA, Fernandez EJ, Manzanera S, Norrby S & Artal P. Adaptive Optics Simulation of Intraocular Lenses with Modified Spherical Aberration. *Invest Ophthalmol Vis Sci.* 2004;45:4601-10.

[150] Marcos S, Barbero S & Jimenez-Alfaro I. Optical Quality and Depth-of-Field of Eyes Implanted with Spherical and Aspheric Intraocular Lenses. *J Refract Surg.* 2005;21:223-35.

[151] Marsack JD, Thibos LN & Applegate RA. Metrics of Optical Quality Derived from Wave Aberrations Predict Visual Performance. *J Vis.* 2004;4:322-8.

[152] Nanavaty MA, Spalton DJ, Boyce J, Saha S & Marshall J. Wavefront Aberrations, Depth of Focus, and Contrast Sensitivity with Aspheric and Spherical Intraocular Lenses: Fellow-Eye Study. *J Cataract Refract Surg.* 2009;35:663-71.

[153] Artigas JM, Menezo JL, Peris C, Felipe A & Diaz-Llopis M. Image Quality with Multifocal Intraocular Lenses and the Effect of Pupil Size: Comparison of Refractive and Hybrid Refractive-Diffractive Designs. *J Cataract Refract Surg.* 2007;33:2111-7.

[154] Guirao A, Redondo M, Geraghty E, et al. Corneal Optical Aberrations and Retinal Image Quality in Patients in Whom Monofocal Intraocular Lenses Were Implanted. *Arch Ophthalmol.* 2002;120:1143-51.

[155] Altmann GE, Nichamin LD, Lane SS & Pepose JS. Optical Performance of 3 Intraocular Lens Designs in the Presence of Decentration. *J Cataract Refract Surg.* 2005;31:574-85.

[156] Rawer R, Stork W, Spraul CW & Lingenfelder C. Imaging Quality of Intraocular Lenses. *J Cataract Refract Surg.* 2005;31:1618-31.

[157] Carkeet A, Velaedan S, Tan YK, Lee DY & Tan DT. Higher Order Ocular Aberrations after Cycloplegic and Non-Cycloplegic Pupil Dilation. *J Refract Surg.* 2003;19:316-22.

[158] Yang Y, Thompson K & Burns SA. Pupil Location under Mesopic, Photopic, and Pharmacologically Dilated Conditions. *Invest Ophthalmol Vis Sci.* 2002;43:2508-12.

[159] Cheng X, Bradley A & Thibos LN. Predicting Subjective Judgment of Best Focus with Objective Image Quality Metrics. *J Vis.* 2004;4:310-21.

[160] Guirao A & Williams DR. A Method to Predict Refractive Errors from Wave Aberration Data. *Optom Vis Sci.* 2003;80:36-42.

[161] Thibos LN. Principles of Hartmann-Shack Aberrometry. *J Refract Surg.* 2000;16:s563-65.

[162] Artal P, Benito A, Perez GM, et al. An Objective Scatter Index Based on Double-Pass Retinal Images of a Point Source to Classify Cataracts. *PLoS One.* 2011;6:e168231-e7.

[163] Vilaseca M, Peris E, Pujol J, Borras R & Arjona M. Intra- and Intersession Repeatability of a Double-Pass Instrument. *Optom Vis Sci.* 2010;87:675-81.
[164] Saad A, Saab M & Gatinel D. Repeatability of Measurements with a Double-Pass System. *J Cataract Refract Surg.* 2010;36:28-33.
[165] Tomas J, Pinero DP & Alio JL. Intra-Observer Repeatability of Optical Quality Measures Provided by a Double-Pass System. *Clin Exp Optom.* 2012;95:60-5.
[166] Ferrer-Blasco T, Garcia-Lazaro S, Montes-Mico R, Cervino A & Gonzalez-Meijome JM. Dynamic Changes in the Air-Tear Film Interface Modulation Transfer Function. *Graefes Arch Clin Exp Ophthalmol.* 2010;248:127-32.
[167] Montes-Mico R, Alio JL, Munoz G & Charman WN. Temporal Changes in Optical Quality of Air-Tear Film Interface at Anterior Cornea after Blink. *Invest Ophthalmol Vis Sci.* 2004;45:1752-7.
[168] Montes-Mico R. Role of the Tear Film in the Optical Quality of the Human Eye. *J Cataract Refract Surg.* 2007;33:1631-5.
[169] Gatinel D. Double Pass-Technique Limitations for Evaluation of Optical Performance after Diffractive IOL Implantation. *J Cataract Refract Surg.* 2011;37:621-2; author reply 2.
[170] Artal P, Marcos S, Navarro R & Williams DR. Odd Aberrations and Double-Pass Measurements of Retinal Image Quality. *J Opt Soc Am A Opt Image Sci Vis.* 1995;12:195-201.
[171] Iglesias I, Berrio E & Artal P. Estimates of the Ocular Wave Aberration from Pairs of Double-Pass Retinal Images. *J Opt Soc Am A Opt Image Sci Vis.* 1998;15:2466-76.
[172] Artal P, Iglesias I, Lopez-Gil N & Green DG. Double-Pass Measurements of the Retinal-Image Quality with Unequal Entrance and Exit Pupil Sizes and the Reversibility of the Eye's Optical System. *J Opt Soc Am A Opt Image Sci Vis.* 1995;12:2358-66.
[173] Iglesias I, Lopez-Gil N & Artal P. Reconstruction of the Point-Spread Function of the Human Eye from Two Double-Pass Retinal Images by Phase-Retrieval Algorithms. *J Opt Soc Am A Opt Image Sci Vis.* 1998;15:326-39.
[174] Diaz-Douton F, Benito A, Pujol J, et al. Comparison of the Retinal Image Quality with a Hartmann-Shack Wavefront Sensor and a Double-Pass Instrument. *Invest Ophthalmol Vis Sci.* 2006;47:1710-6.

[175] Rodriguez P & Navarro R. Double-Pass Versus Aberrometric Modulation Transfer Function in Green Light. *J Biomed Opt.* 2007;12:044018.
[176] Cazal J, Lavin-Dapena C, Marin J & Verges C. Accommodative Intraocular Lens Tilting. *Am J Ophthalmol.* 2005;140:341-4.
[177] Taketani F, Matuura T, Yukawa E & Hara Y. Influence of Intraocular Lens Tilt and Decentration on Wavefront Aberrations. *J Cataract Refract Surg.* 2004;30:2158-62.
[178] Patel CK, Ormonde S, Rosen PH & Bron AJ. Postoperative Intraocular Lens Rotation: A Randomized Comparison of Plate and Loop Haptic Implants. *Ophthalmology.* 1999;106:2190-5; discussion 6.
[179] Vass C, Menapace R, Schmetterer K, et al. Prediction of Pseudophakic Capsular Bag Diameter Based on Biometric Variables. *J Cataract Refract Surg.* 1999;25:1376-81.
[180] Shimizu K, Misawa A & Suzuki Y. Toric Intraocular Lenses: Correcting Astigmatism While Controlling Axis Shift. *J Cataract Refract Surg.* 1994;20:523-6.
[181] Chang DF. Comparative Rotational Stability of Single-Piece Open-Loop Acrylic and Plate-Haptic Silicone Toric Intraocular Lenses. *J Cataract Refract Surg.* 2008;34:1842-7.
[182] Chua WH, Yuen LH, Chua J, Teh G & Hill WE. Matched Comparison of Rotational Stability of 1-Piece Acrylic and Plate-Haptic Silicone Toric Intraocular Lenses in Asian Eyes. *J Cataract Refract Surg.* 2012;38:620-4.
[183] Oshika T, Nagata T & Ishii Y. Adhesion of Lens Capsule to Intraocular Lenses of Polymethylmethacrylate, Silicone, and Acrylic Foldable Materials: An Experimental Study. *Br J Ophthalmol.* 1998;82:549-53.
[184] Gerten G, Michels A & Olmes A. [Toric Intraocular Lenses. Clinical Results and Rotational Stability]. *Ophthalmologe.* 2001;98:715-20.
[185] Shah GD, Praveen MR, Vasavada AR, et al. Rotational Stability of a Toric Intraocular Lens: Influence of Axial Length and Alignment in the Capsular Bag. *J Cataract Refract Surg.* 2012;38:54-9.
[186] Zuberbuhler B, Signer T, Gale R & Haefliger E. Rotational Stability of the AcrySof SA60TT Toric Intraocular Lenses: A Cohort Study. *BMC Ophthalmology.* 2008;8:1-5.
[187] Mendicute J, Irigoyen C, Ruiz M, et al. Toric Intraocular Lens Versus Opposite Clear Corneal Incisions to Correct Astigmatism in Eyes Having Cataract Surgery. *J Cataract Refract Surg.* 2009;35:451-8.

[188] De Silva DJ, Ramkissoon YD & Bloom PA. Evaluation of a Toric Intraocular Lens with a Z-Haptic. *J Cataract Refract Surg.* 2006;32:1492-8.
[189] Chang DF. Early Rotational Stability of the Longer STAAR Toric Intraocular Lens: Fifty Consecutive Cases. *J Cataract Refract Surg.* 2003;29:935-40.
[190] Jampaulo M, Olson MD & Miller KM. Long-Term STAAR Toric Intraocular Lens Rotational Stability. *Am J Ophthalmol.* 2008;146:550-3.
[191] Kim MH, Chung TY & Chung ES. Long-Term Efficacy and Rotational Stability of AcrySof Toric Intraocular Lens Implantation in Cataract Surgery. *Korean J Ophthalmol.* 2010;24:207-12.
[192] Koshy JJ, Nishi Y, Hirnschall N, et al. Rotational Stability of a Single-Piece Toric Acrylic Intraocular Lens. *J Cataract Refract Surg.* 2010;36:1665-70.
[193] Wolffsohn JS & Buckhurst PJ. Objective Analysis of Toric Intraocular Lens Rotation and Centration. *J Cataract Refract Surg.* 2010;36:778-82.
[194] Visser N, Berendschot TT, Bauer NJ, et al. Accuracy of Toric Intraocular Lens Implantation in Cataract and Refractive Surgery. *J Cataract Refract Surg.* 2011;37:1394-402.
[195] Weinand F, Jung A, Stein A, et al. Rotational Stability of a Single-Piece Hydrophobic Acrylic Intraocular Lens: New Method for High-Precision Rotation Control. *J Cataract Refract Surg.* 2007;33:800 - 3.
[196] Sasaki K, Sakamoto Y, Shibata T, Nakaizumi H & Emori Y. Measurement of Postoperative Intraocular Lens Tilting and Decentration Using Scheimpflug Images. *J Cataract Refract Surg.* 1989;15:454-7.
[197] Jung CK, Chung SK & Baek NH. Decentration and Tilt: Silicone Multifocal Versus Acrylic Soft Intraocular Lenses. *J Cataract Refract Surg.* 2000;26:582-5.
[198] Hayashi K, Hayashi H, Nakao F & Hayashi F. Comparison of Decentration and Tilt between One Piece and Three Piece Polymethyl Methacrylate Intraocular Lenses. *Br J Ophthalmol.* 1998;82:419-22.
[199] Hayashi K, Harada M, Hayashi H, Nakao F & Hayashi F. Decentration and Tilt of Polymethyl Methacrylate, Silicone, and Acrylic Soft Intraocular Lenses. *Ophthalmology.* 1997;104:793-8.
[200] Hayashi K, Hayashi H, Nakao F & Hayashi F. Intraocular Lens Tilt and Decentration, Anterior Chamber Depth, and Refractive Error after Trans-Scleral Suture Fixation Surgery. *Ophthalmology.* 1999;106:878-82.

[201] Rosales P, Dubbelman M, Marcos S & van der Heijde R. Crystalline Lens Radii of Curvature from Purkinje and Scheimpflug Imaging. *J Vis.* 2006;6:1057-67.
[202] Rosales P & Marcos S. Pentacam Scheimpflug Quantitative Imaging of the Crystalline Lens and Intraocular Lens. *J Refract Surg.* 2009;25:421-8.
[203] de Castro A, Rosales P & Marcos S. Tilt and Decentration of Intraocular Lenses In-Vivo from Purkinje and Scheimpflug Imaging. Validation Study. *J Cataract Refract Surg.* 2007;33:418-29.
[204] Drews RC. Depth of Field in Slit Lamp Photography. An Optical Solution Using the Scheimpflug Principle. *Ophthalmologica.* 1964;148:143-50.
[205] Wolffsohn JS & Davies LN. Advances in Ocular Imaging. *Expert Rev Ophthalmol.* 2007;2:755-67.
[206] Fink W. Refractive Correction Method for Digital Charge-Coupled Device-Recorded Scheimpflug Photographs by Means of Ray Tracing. *J Biomed Opt.* 2005;10:024003.
[207] Patel S, Alio JL & Perez-Santonja JJ. A Model to Explain the Difference Between Changes in Refraction and Central Ocular Surface Power after Laser in Situ Keratomileusis. *J Refract Surg.* 2000;16:330-5.
[208] Oshika T, Kawana K, Hiraoka T, Kaji Y & Kiuchi T. Ocular Higher-Order Wavefront Aberration Caused by Major Tilting of Intraocular Lens. *Am J Ophthalmol.* 2005;140:744-6.
[209] Viestenz A, Seitz B & Langenbucher A. Evaluating the Eye's Rotational Stability During Standard Photography. Effect on Determining the Axial Orientation of Toric Intraocular Lenses. *J Cataract Refract Surg.* 2005;31:557-61.
[210] Nishi Y, Hirnschall N, Crnej A, et al. Reproducibility of Intraocular Lens Decentration and Tilt Measurement Using a Clinical Purkinje Meter. *J Cataract Refract Surg.* 2010;36:1529-35.
[211] Tabernero J, Benito A, Nourrit V & Artal P. Instrument for Measuring the Misalignments of Ocular Surfaces. *Opt Express.* 2006;14:10945-56.
[212] Tabernero J, Piers P, Benito A, Redondo M & Artal P. Predicting the Optical Performance of Eyes Implanted with IOLs to Correct Spherical Aberration. *Invest Ophthalmol Vis Sci.* 2006;47:4651-8.
[213] Rosales P & Marcos S. Phakometry and Lens Tilt and Decentration Using a Custom-Developed Purkinje Imaging Apparatus: Validation and Measurements. *J Opt Soc Am A Opt Image Sci Vis.* 2006;23:509-20.

[214] Shoji N & Shimizu K. Binocular Function of the Patient with the Refractive Multifocal Intraocular Lens. *J Cataract Refract Surg.* 2002;28:1012-7.
[215] Ferrer-Blasco T, Madrid-Costa D, Garcia-Lazaro S, Cervino A & Montes-Mico R. Stereopsis in Bilaterally Multifocal Pseudophakic Patients. *Graefes Arch Clin Exp Ophthalmol.* 2011;249:245-51.
[216] Arens B, Freudenthaler N & Quentin CD. Binocular Function after Bilateral Implantation of Monofocal and Refractive Multifocal Intraocular Lenses. *J Cataract Refract Surg.* 1999;25:399-404.
[217] Jacobi FK, Kammann J, Jacobi KW, Grosskopf U & Walden K. Bilateral Implantation of Asymmetrical Diffractive Multifocal Intraocular Lenses. *Arch Ophthalmol.* 1999;117:17-23.
[218] Boberg-Ans J. Differences and Similarities in a Series of Cases with Bilateral Intraocular Lenses and Evaluation of the Results. *Br J Ophthalmol.* 1977;61:622-7.
[219] Hayashi K & Hayashi H. Stereopsis in Bilaterally Pseudophakic Patients. *J Cataract Refract Surg.* 2004;30:1466-70.
[220] Jacobi PC, Dietlein TS, Lueke C & Jacobi FK. Multifocal Intraocular Lens Implantation in Patients with Traumatic Cataract. *Ophthalmology.* 2003;110:531-8.
[221] Haring G, Gronemeyer A, Hedderich J & de Decker W. Stereoacuity and Aniseikonia after Unilateral and Bilateral Implantation of the Array Refractive Multifocal Intraocular Lens. *J Cataract Refract Surg.* 1999;25:1151-6.
[222] Nourrit V & Kelly JMF. Intraocular Scatter and Visual Performances. *Optom Pract.* 2009;10:117-28.
[223] Vos JJ. Disability Glare—a State of the Art Report. *CIE Journal.* 1984; 3:39-53.
[224] IJspeert JK, de Waard PW, van den Berg TJ & de Jong PT. The Intraocular Straylight Function in 129 Healthy Volunteers; Dependence on Angle, Age and Pigmentation. *Vision Res.* 1990;30:699-707.
[225] Coppens JE, Franssen L, van Rijn LJ & van den Berg TJ. Reliability of the Compensation Comparison Stray-Light Measurement Method. *J Biomed Opt.* 2006;11:0340271-9.
[226] Franssen L, Coppens JE & van den Berg TJ. Compensation Comparison Method for Assessment of Retinal Straylight. *Invest Ophthalmol Vis Sci.* 2006;47:768-76.
[227] Cervino A, Montes-Mico R & Hosking SL. Performance of the Compensation Comparison Method for Retinal Straylight Measurement:

Effect of Patient's Age on Repeatability. *Br J Ophthalmol.* 2008;92:788-91.
[228] Holladay JT, Van Dijk H, Lang A, et al. Optical Performance of Multifocal Intraocular Lenses. *J Cataract Refract Surg.* 1990;16:413-22.
[229] Davison JA & Simpson MJ. History and Development of the Apodized Diffractive Intraocular Lens. *J Cataract Refract Surg.* 2006;32:849-58.
[230] Hofmann T, Zuberbuhler B, Cervino A, Montes-Mico R & Haefliger E. Retinal Straylight and Complaint Scores 18 Months after Implantation of the AcrySof Monofocal and ReSTOR Diffractive Intraocular Lenses. *J Refract Surg.* 2009;25:485-92.
[231] Visser N, Nuijts RM, de Vries NE & Bauer NJ. Visual Outcomes and Patient Satisfaction after Cataract Surgery with Toric Multifocal Intraocular Lens Implantation. *J Cataract Refract Surg.* 2011;37:2034-42.
[232] Cervino A, Hosking SL, Montes-Mico R & Alio JL. Retinal Straylight in Patients with Monofocal and Multifocal Intraocular Lenses. *J Cataract Refract Surg.* 2008;34:441-6.
[233] de Vries NE, Franssen L, Webers CA, et al. Intraocular Straylight after Implantation of the Multifocal AcrySof ReSTOR SA60D3 Diffractive Intraocular Lens. *J Cataract Refract Surg.* 2008;34:957-62.
[234] Pieh S, Lackner B, Hanselmayer G, et al. Halo Size under Distance and near Conditions in Refractive Multifocal Intraocular Lenses. *Br J Ophthalmol.* 2001;85:816-21.
[235] Dick HB, Krummenauer F, Schwenn O, Krist R & Pfeiffer N. Objective and Subjective Evaluation of Photic Phenomena after Monofocal and Multifocal Intraocular Lens Implantation. *Ophthalmology.* 1999;106:1878-86.
[236] Buckhurst PJ, Wolffsohn JS, Shah S, Naroo S & Davies LN. Evaluation of Dysphotopsia with Multifocal Intraocular Lenses. *Invest Ophthalmol Vis Sci.* 2011;52:(E-Abstract 6185).
[237] Lundstrom M & Pesudovs K. Questionnaires for Measuring Cataract Surgery Outcomes. *J Cataract Refract Surg.* 2011;37:945-59.
[238] McAlinden C, Gothwal VK, Khadka J, et al. A Head-to-Head Comparison of 16 Cataract Surgery Outcome Questionnaires. *Ophthalmology.* 2011;118:2374-81.
[239] Javitt JC, Wang F, Trentacost DJ, Rowe M & Tarantino N. Outcomes of Cataract Extraction with Multifocal Intraocular Lens Implantation: Functional Status and Quality of Life. *Ophthalmology.* 1997;104:589-99.

[240] Javitt JC, Jacobson G & Schiffman RM. Validity and Reliability of the Cataract Type Spec: An Instrument for Measuring Outcomes of Cataract Extraction. *Am J Ophthalmol.* 2003;136:285-90.
[241] Gothwal VK, Wright TA, Lamoureux EL & Pesudovs K. Using Rasch Analysis to Revisit the Validity of the Cataract Type Spec Instrument for Measuring Cataract Surgery Outcomes. *J Cataract Refract Surg.* 2009;35:1509-17.
[242] Rasch G. On General Laws and the Meaning of Measurement in Psychology. In: Neyman J, editor. *Proceedings of the 4th Berkeley Symposium on Mathematical Statistics and Probability*; 1961; Berkeley, California: University of California Press; 1961. p. 321-34.
[243] Gupta N, Wolffsohn JS, Naroo SA, et al. Development of a Near Activity Visual Questionnaire to Assess Accommodating Intraocular Lenses. *Cont Lens Anterior Eye.* 2007;30:134-43.
[244] Buckhurst PJ, Wolffsohn JS, Gupta N, et al. Development of a Questionnaire to Assess the Relative Subjective Benefits of Presbyopia Correction. *J Cataract Refract Surg.* 2012;38:74-9.
[245] McAlinden C, Pesudovs K & Moore JE. The Development of an Instrument to Measure Quality of Vision: The Quality of Vision (QoV) Questionnaire. *Invest Ophthalmol Vis Sci.* 2010;51:5537-45.
[246] Steinberg EP, Tielsch JM, Schein OD, et al. The VF-14. An Index of Functional Impairment in Patients with Cataract. *Arch Ophthalmol.* 1994;112:630-8.
[247] Alonso J, Espallargues M, Andersen TF, et al. International Applicability of the VF-14. An Index of Visual Function in Patients with Cataracts. *Ophthalmology.* 1997;104:799-807.
[248] Brydon KW, Tokarewicz AC & Nichols BD. AMO Array Multifocal Lens Versus Monofocal Correction in Cataract Surgery. *J Cataract Refract Surg.* 2000;26:96-100.
[249] Nijkamp MD, Dolders MG, de Brabander J, et al. Effectiveness of Multifocal Intraocular Lenses to Correct Presbyopia after Cataract Surgery: A Randomized Controlled Trial. *Ophthalmology.* 2004;111:1832-9.
[250] Uusitalo RJ, Brans T, Pessi T & Tarkkanen A. Evaluating Cataract Surgery Gains by Assessing Patients' Quality of Life Using the VF-7. *J Cataract Refract Surg.* 1999;25:989-94.
[251] Sen HN, Sarikkola AU, Uusitalo RJ & Laatikainen L. Quality of Vision after AMO Array Multifocal Intraocular Lens Implantation. *J Cataract Refract Surg.* 2004;30:2483-93.

[252] Gothwal VK, Wright TA, Lamoureux EL & Pesudovs K. Measuring Outcomes of Cataract Surgery Using the Visual Function Index-14. *J Cataract Refract Surg.* 2010;36:1181-8.

[253] Lundstrom M, Roos P, Jensen S & Fregell G. Catquest Questionnaire for Use in Cataract Surgery Care: Description, Validity, and Reliability. *J Cataract Refract Surg.* 1997;23:1226-36.

[254] Lundstrom M, Stenevi U, Thorburn W & Roos P. Catquest Questionnaire for Use in Cataract Surgery Care: Assessment of Surgical Outcomes. *J Cataract Refract Surg.* 1998;24:968-74.

[255] Lundstrom M & Pesudovs K. Catquest-9SF Patient Outcomes Questionnaire: Nine-Item Short-Form Rasch-Scaled Revision of the Catquest Questionnaire. *J Cataract Refract Surg.* 2009;35:504-13.

[256] Mangione CM, Lee PP, Pitts J, et al. Psychometric Properties of the National Eye Institute Visual Function Questionnaire (Nei-Vfq). *Arch Ophthalmol.* 1998;116:1496-504.

[257] Mangione CM, Lee PP, Gutierrez PR, et al. Development of the 25-Item National Eye Institute Visual Function Questionnaire. *Arch Ophthalmol.* 2001;119:1050-8.

[258] Kohnen T, Nuijts R, Levy P, Haefliger E & Alfonso JF. Visual Function after Bilateral Implantation of Apodized Diffractive Aspheric Multifocal Intraocular Lenses with a +3.0 D Addition. *J Cataract Refract Surg.* 2009;35:2062-9.

[259] Munoz G, Albarran-Diego C, Ferrer-Blasco T, Sakla HF & Garcia-Lazaro S. Visual Function after Bilateral Implantation of a New Zonal Refractive Aspheric Multifocal Intraocular Lens. *J Cataract Refract Surg.* 2011;37:2043-52.

[260] Donovan JL, Brookes ST, Laidlaw DA, et al. The Development and Validation of a Questionnaire to Assess Visual Symptoms/Dysfunction and Impact on Quality of Life in Cataract Patients: The Visual Symptoms and Quality of Life (VSQ) Questionnaire. *Ophthalmic Epidemiol.* 2003;10:49-65.

[261] Chiam PJ, Chan JH, Aggarwal RK & Kasaby S. ReSTOR Intraocular Lens Implantation in Cataract Surgery: Quality of Vision. *J Cataract Refract Surg.* 2006;32:1459-63.

[262] Haring G, Dick HB, Krummenauer F, Weissmantel U & Kroncke W. Subjective Photic Phenomena with Refractive Multifocal and Monofocal Intraocular Lenses. Results of a Multicenter Questionnaire. *J Cataract Refract Surg.* 2001;27:245-9.

[263] Wallin TR, Hinckley M, Nilson C & Olson RJ. A Clinical Comparison of Single-Piece and Three-Piece Truncated Hydrophobic Acrylic Intraocular Lenses. *Am J Ophthalmol.* 2003;136:614-9.
[264] Tester R, Pace NL, Samore M & Olson RJ. Dysphotopsia in Phakic and Pseudophakic Patients: Incidence and Relation to Intraocular Lens Type(2). *J Cataract Refract Surg.* 2000;26:810-6.
[265] Massof RW. The Measurement of Vision Disability. *Optom Vis Sci.* 2002;79:516-52.
[266] Food & Drug Administration. Guidance for Industry; *Patient-Reported Outcome Measures: Use in Medical Product Development to Support Labeling Claims Webpage* 2009 [cited 11th June 2011]; Available from:http://www.fda.gov/downloads/Drugs/GuidanceCompliance RegulatoryInformation/Guidances/UCM193282.pdf
[267] Schaumberg DA, Dana MR, Christen WG & Glynn RJ. A Systematic Overview of the Incidence of Posterior Capsule Opacification. *Ophthalmology.* 1998;105:1213-21.
[268] Nagata T & Watanabe I. Optic Sharp Edge or Convexity: Comparison of Effects on Posterior Capsular Opacification. *Jpn J Ophthalmol.* 1996;40:397-403.
[269] Kruger AJ, Schauersberger J, Abela C, Schild G & Amon M. Two Year Results: Sharp Versus Rounded Optic Edges on Silicone Lenses. *J Cataract Refract Surg.* 2000;26:566-70.
[270] Sellman TR & Lindstrom RL. Effect of a Plano-Convex Posterior Chamber Lens on Capsular Opacification from Elschnig Pearl Formation. *J Cataract Refract Surg.* 1988;14:68-72.
[271] Findl O, Buehl W, Menapace R, et al. Comparison of 4 Methods for Quantifying Posterior Capsule Opacification. *J Cataract Refract Surg.* 2003;29:106-11.
[272] Hayashi K, Hayashi H, Nakao F & Hayashi F. In-Vivo Quantitative Measurement of Posterior Capsule Opacification after Extracapsular Cataract Surgery. *Am J Ophthalmol.* 1998;125:837-43.
[273] Lasa MS, Datiles MB, 3rd, Magno BV & Mahurkar A. Scheimpflug Photography and Postcataract Surgery Posterior Capsule Opacification. *Ophthalmic Surg.* 1995;26:110-3.
[274] Grewal D, Jain R, Brar GS & Grewal SP. Pentacam Tomograms: A Novel Method for Quantification of Posterior Capsule Opacification. *Invest Ophthalmol Vis Sci.* 2008;49:2004-8.

[275] Aslam TM, Dhillon B, Werghi N, Taguri A & Wadood A. Systems of Analysis of Posterior Capsule Opacification. *Br J Ophthalmol.* 2002;86:1181-6.
[276] Wang MC & Woung LC. Digital Retroilluminated Photography to Analyze Posterior Capsule Opacification in Eyes with Intraocular Lenses. *J Cataract Refract Surg.* 2000;26:56-61.
[277] Camparini M, Macaluso C, Reggiani L & Maraini G. Retroillumination Versus Reflected-Light Images in the Photographic Assessment of Posterior Capsule Opacification. *Invest Ophthalmol Vis Sci.* 2000;41:3074-9.
[278] Pande MV, Ursell PG, Spalton DJ, Heath G & Kundaiker S. High-Resolution Digital Retroillumination Imaging of the Posterior Lens Capsule after Cataract Surgery. *J Cataract Refract Surg.* 1997;23:1521-7.
[279] Friedman DS, Duncan DD, Munoz B, West SK & Schein OD. Digital Image Capture and Automated Analysis of Posterior Capsular Opacification. *Invest Ophthalmol Vis Sci.* 1999;40:1715-26.
[280] Tetz MR & Nimsgern C. Posterior Capsule Opacification. Part 2: Clinical Findings. *J Cataract Refract Surg.* 1999;25:1662-74.
[281] Barman SA, Hollick EJ, Boyce JF, et al. Quantification of Posterior Capsular Opacification in Digital Images after Cataract Surgery. *Invest Ophthalmol Vis Sci.* 2000;41:3882-92.
[282] Bender L, Spalton DJ, Uyanonvara B, et al. POCOman: New System for Quantifying Posterior Capsule Opacification. *J Cataract Refract Surg.* 2004;30:2058-63.
[283] Buehl W, Findl O, Menapace R, et al. Reproducibility of Standardized Retroillumination Photography for Quantification of Posterior Capsule Opacification. *J Cataract Refract Surg.* 2002;28:265-70.
[284] Sacu S, Menapace R, Findl O, et al. Long-Term Efficacy of Adding a Sharp Posterior Optic Edge to a Three-Piece Silicone Intraocular Lens on Capsule Opacification: Five-Year Results of a Randomized Study. *Am J Ophthalmol.* 2005;139:696-703.
[285] Bohorquez V & Alarcon R. Long-Term Reading Performance in Patients with Bilateral Dual-Optic Accommodating Intraocular Lenses. *J Cataract Refract Surg.* 2010;36:1880-6.
[286] Tahzib NG, Nuijts RM, Wu WY & Budo CJ. Long-Term Study of Artisan Phakic Intraocular Lens Implantation for the Correction of Moderate to High Myopia: Ten-Year Follow-up Results. *Ophthalmology.* 2007;114:1133-42.

[287] Hauranieh N & Giardini P. A High-Tech New Device Eyevispod Helps to Evlauate Refractive Lens Surgery and Other Presbyopic Surgeries on near and Intermediate Vision Quality. *Eur Ophthal Rev.* 2011;5:46-9.

In: Cataracts and Cataract Surgery
Editor: Didier Navarro

ISBN: 978-1-62808-400-9
© 2013 Nova Science Publishers, Inc.

Chapter II

Cataracts: Epidemiology, Morphology, Types and Risk Factors

Dieudonne Kaimbo Wa Kaimbo[*]
Department of Ophthalmology, University of Kinshasa
Democratic Republic of Congo

Abstract

Cataract is the leading cause of blindness (defined as visual acuity less than 20/400) worldwide and is responsible for approximately 50% of the estimated 40 million cases of blindness in the developing world. In the next 20 years there will be doubling of cataract visual morbidity. Oxidation of lens proteins and mitochondrial function are key factors in cataract pathogenesis. This chapter focuses on epidemiology, morphology and different types of cataracts. The chapter also presents a comprehensive overview of specific and general cataract risk factors. Contents based on recent findings published in the medical literature and will reflect the most advanced achievements in current clinical and experimental research on cataracts.

---

[*] Corresponding author: E-mail: dieudonne_kaimbo@yahoo.com.

1. Epidemiology

Cataract is the leading cause of blindness and visual impairment throughout the *world, according to* the World Health Organization (WHO) (Ressnikoff et al, 2004). With the general aging of the population, the overall prevalence of vision loss as a result of lenticular opacities increases each year. In 2002, the WHO estimated that cataracts caused reversible blindness in more than 17 million (47.8%) of the 37 million blind individuals worldwide, and this number is projected to reach 40 million by 2020.

In England and the United States the prevalence of cataract in the general population aged 45 to 64 years is between 2 and 8%, rising to between 21 and 39% in the 65 to 75 year age group, and to 65% in those aged 85 years and over (Leibowitz et al, 1980; Klein and Klein, 1982; Gibson et al, 1985). In the Framingham Eye Study from 1973-1975, senile cataract was seen in 15.5% of the 2477 patients examined. The overall rates of senile cataract in general, and of its 3 main types (ie, nuclear, cortical, posterior subcapsular), rapidly increased with age; for the oldest age group ($\geq$ 75 y), nuclear, cortical, and posterior subcapsular cataracts were found in 65.5%, 27.7%, and 19.7% of the study population, respectively. Nuclear opacities were the most commonly seen lens change. An updated study by the Wilmer Eye Institute in 2004 noted that approximately 20.5 million (17.2%) Americans older than 40 years had a cataract in either eye or 6.1 million (5.1%) were pseudophakic/aphakic (Congdon et al, 2004).These numbers are expected to rise to 30.1 million cataracts and 9.5 million cases with pseudophakia/aphakia by 2020.

Prevent Blindness America currently estimates that more than 22 million Americans aged 40 years and older have a cataract. An average of 3 million Americans undergo cataract surgery every year, with a 95% success rate of obtaining a best corrected vision of 20/20-20/40. An analysis of blind registration forms in the west of Scotland showed senile cataract as 1 of the 4 leading causes of blindness.

In recent studies done in China (Liang et al, 2008; You et al, 2011), Canada (Maberley and Hollands, 2006), Japan (Iwase et al, 2006), Denmark (Buch et al, 2001), Argentina (Limburg et al, 2008), and India (Murthy et al, 2010), cataract was identified as the leading cause of visual impairment and blindness, with statistics ranging from 33.3% (Denmark) to as high as 82.6% (India). Published data estimate that 1.2% of the entire population of Africa is blind, with cataract causing 36% of this blindness. In a survey conducted in 3 districts in the Punjab plains, the overall rates of occurrence of senile cataract was 15.3% among 1269 persons examined who were aged 30 years and older and 4.3% for all ages. This increased markedly to 67% for ages 70 years and older.

Studies have found racial differences in the prevalence of different cataract types. In the Salisbury Eye Evaluation Study, Americans of African descent had a four times greater chance of having cortical opacities than Americans of European descent, and Americans of European descent were more likely to have nuclear and PSC opacities (West et al, 1998). The Los Angeles Latino Eye Study of individuals 40 years old or older found that cortical opacities were the most frequent type of lens opacity (Varma and Torres, 2004).

A follow-up to the Beaver Dam Eye Study was performed between 1993 and 1995 to estimate the incidence of nuclear, cortical, and posterior subcapsular cataract (PSC) in the study cohort. Incident nuclear cataract occurred in 13.1% of the study cohort, cortical cataract in 8.2%, and posterior subcapsular cataract (PSC) in 3.4%. The cumulative incidence of nuclear cataract increased from 2.9% in persons aged 43–54 years at baseline to 40.0% in those aged 75 years or older. For cortical cataract and PSC, the corresponding values were 1.9% and 21.8% and 1.4% and 7.3%, respectively. Women were more likely than men to have nuclear cataracts, even after adjustments for age were made (AAO, 2011).

There is evidence that genetics plays a role in the formation of cataract, especially congenital cataract (Kannabiran, 2000). Congenital cataract is a significant cause of visual impairment or blindness in childhood. The prevalence of congenital cataracts is 1 to 6 per 10,000 live births, depending on the ascertainment method (Holmes et al, 2003). Globally, congenital cataracts account for nearly one tenth of childhood blindness from different causes including infections during embryogenesis, metabolic disorders (galactosemia), and genetic defects (Reddy et al, 2004). Statistical analyses have revealed that about one quarter of congenital cataracts are hereditary (Amaya et al, 2003). Genetically, the majority of isolated congenital cataracts exhibit as autosomal dominant, although autosomal recessive and X-linked inherited forms have also been reported (Vanita et al, 1999). Currently, there are more than 40 genetic loci to which isolated or primary cataracts have been mapped, and more than 26 genes have been characterized, although this number is constantly increasing (Shiels and Hejtmancik, 2007). The crystallin and connexin genes appear to be the most commonly associated with congenital cataract.

2. Morphology

Cataracts may be partial or complete, stationary or progressive, or hard or soft. There are many morphological types of cataracts. Morphologic types include:

2.1. Age-Related Lens Changes

As the lens ages, it increases in mass and thickness and decreases in accommodative power. As new layers of cortical fibers form concentrically, the lens nucleus undergoes compression and hardening (nuclear sclerosis). Chemical modification and proteolytic cleavage of crystallins (lens proteins) result in the formation of high-molecular-mass protein aggregates. These aggregates may become large enough to cause abrupt fluctuations in the local refractive index of the lens, thereby scattering light and reducing transparency. Chemical modification of lens nuclear proteins also increases pigmentation, such that the lens becomes increasingly yellow or brown with advancing age. Other age-related changes include decreased concentrations of glutathione and potassium and increased concentrations of sodium and calcium in the lens cell cytoplasm (American Academy of Ophthalmology (AAO), 2011).

A very common cause of visual impairment in older adults is age-related cataract, the pathogenesis of which is multifactorial and not completely understood. There are 3 main types of age-related cataracts: nuclear, cortical, and posterior subcapsular. In many patients, components of more than one type are present.

Nuclear Cataracts

Some degree of nuclear sclerosis and yellowing is normal in adult patients after the age of 50. In general, this condition interferes only minimally with visual function. An excessive amount of light scattering and yellowing is called a nuclear cataract, which causes a central opacity. The ophthalmologist can evaluate the degree of increased color and of opacification by using a slit-lamp biomicroscope and by examining the red reflex with the pupil dilated.

Nuclear cataracts tend to progress slowly. Although they are usually bilateral, they may be asymmetric. Nuclear cataracts typically cause greater impairment of distance vision than of near vision. In the early stages, the progressive hardening of the lens nucleus frequently causes an increase in the refractive index of the lens and thus a myopic shift in refraction (lenticular myopia). In hyperopic eyes, the myopic shift enables otherwise presbyopic individuals to read without spectacles, a condition referred to as 'second sight of the aged'. Occasionally, the abrupt change in refractive index between the sclerotic nucleus (or other lens opacities) and the lens cortex can cause monocular diplopia. Progressive yellowing or browning of the lens causes patients to have poor color discrimination, especially at the blue end of the visible light spectrum. Photopic retinal function may decrease with advanced nuclear cataract. In very advanced cases, the lens nucleus becomes opaque and brown and is called a brunescent nuclear cataract (AAO, 2011).

Histologically, the nucleus in nuclear cataract is difficult to distinguish from the nucleus of normal, aged lenses. Investigations by electron microscopy have identified an increased number of lamellar membrane whorls in some nuclear cataracts. The degree to which protein aggregates or these membrane modifications contribute to the increased light scattering of nuclear cataracts is unclear (AAO, 2011).

Cortical Cataracts

In contrast to nuclear cataracts, cortical cataracts are associated with the local disruption of the structure of mature lens fiber cells. Once membrane integrity is compromised, essential metabolites are lost from the affected cells. This loss leads to extensive protein oxidation and precipitation. Cortical cataracts are usually bilateral but are often asymmetric. Their effect on visual function varies greatly, depending on the location of the opacification relative to the visual axis. A common symptom of cortical cataracts is glare from intense focal light sources, such as car headlights. Monocular diplopia may also result. Cortical cataracts vary greatly in their rate of progression, with some cortical opacities remaining unchanged for prolonged periods and others progressing rapidly.

The first signs of cortical cataract formation visible with the slit-lamp biomicroscope are vacuoles and water clefts in the anterior or posterior cortex. The cortical lamellae may be separated by fluid. Wedge-shaped opacities (often called cortical spokes or cuneiform opacities) form near the periphery of the lens, with the pointed end of the opacities oriented toward the center. Since these peripheral opacities occur in fiber cells that extend from the posterior to the anterior sutures, they affect only the equatorial regions of the fiber cells. In the initial stages of the cataract, affected fiber cells remain clear at their anterior and posterior ends. The cortical spokes appear as white opacities when viewed with the slit-lamp biomicroscope and as dark shadows when viewed on retroillumination. The wedge-shaped opacities may spread to adjacent fiber cells and along the length of affected fibers, causing the degree of opacity to increase and extend toward the visual axis. When the entire cortex from the capsule to the nucleus becomes white and opaque, the cataract is said to be mature. In mature opacities, the lens takes up water, swelling to become an intumescent cortical cataract (AAO, 2011).

When degenerated cortical material leaks through the lens capsule, leaving the capsule wrinkled and shrunken, the cataract is referred to as hypermature. When further liquefaction of the cortex allows free movement of the nucleus within the capsular bag, the term morgagnian cataract is used (AAO, 2011).

Histologically, cortical cataracts are characterized by local swelling and disruption of the lens fiber cells. Globules of eosinophilic material (morgagnian globules) are observed in slitlike spaces between lens fibers (AAO, 2011).

Posterior Subcapsular Cataracts

Posterior subcapsular cataracts (PSCs) are often seen in patients younger than those presenting with nuclear or cortical cataracts. PSCs are located in the posterior cortical layer and are usually axial. The first indication of PSC formation is a subtle iridescent sheen in the posterior cortical layers visible with the slit lamp. In later stages, granular opacities and a plaquelike opacity of the posterior subcapsular cortex appear (AAO, 2011).

The patient often complains of glare and poor vision under bright lighting conditions because the PSC obscures more of the pupillary aperture when miosis is induced by bright lights, accommodation, or miotics. Near vision tends to be reduced more than distance vision. Some patients experience monocular diplopia. Slit-lamp detection of PSCs can best be accomplished through a dilated pupil. Retroillumination is also helpful.

As stated earlier, PSCs are one of the main types of cataract related to aging. However, they can also occur as a result of trauma; systemic, topical, or intraocular corticosteroid use; inflammation; exposure to ionizing radiation; and alcoholism (AAO, 20211).

Histologically, PSC is associated with posterior migration of the lens epithelial cells from the lens equator to the visual axis on the inner surface of the posterior capsule. During their migration to or after their arrival at the posterior axis, the cells undergo aberrant enlargement. These swollen cells are called Wedl, or bladder, cells (AAO, 2011).

2.2. Traumatic Cataracts

Trauma is the most common cause of unilateral cataract in young individuals.Traumatic lens damage may be caused by mechanical injury and by physical forces (radiation, chemicals, electrical current).

Contusion

Vossius Ring

Blunt injury to the eye can sometimes cause a ring of pigment from the pupillary ruff to be imprinted on the anterior surface of the lens; this is referred to as a Vossius ring. Although a Vossius ring is visually insignificant and gradually resolves with time, it serves as an indicator of prior blunt trauma

Traumatic Cataract

A blunt, nonperforating injury may cause lens opacification either as an acute event or as a late sequela. A contusion cataract may involve only a portion of the lens or the entire lens. Often, the initial manifestation of a contusion cataract is a stellate or rosette-shaped opacification (rosette cataract), usually axial in location, that involves the posterior lens capsule. In some cases, blunt trauma causes both dislocation and cataract formation. Mild contusion cataracts can improve spontaneously in rare cases (AAO, 2011).

Dislocation and Subluxation

During a blunt injury to the eye, rapid expansion of the globe in an equatorial plane immediately follows compression. This rapid equatorial expansion can disrupt the zonular fibers, causing dislocation or subluxation of the lens. The lens may be dislocated in any direction, including posteriorly into the vitreous cavity or anteriorly into the anterior chamber (Irvine and Smith, 1991).

Symptoms and signs of traumatic lens subluxation include fluctuation of vision, impaired accommodation, monocular diplopia, and high astigmatism. Often, iridodonesis or phacodonesis is present. Retroillumination of the lens at the slit lamp through a dilated pupil may reveal the zonular disruption. In some cases, blunt trauma causes both dislocation and cataract formation (Irvine and Smith, 1991).

Perforating and Penetrating Injury

A perforating or penetrating injury of the lens often results in opacification of the cortex at the site of the rupture, usually progressing rapidly to complete opacification. Occasionally, a small perforating injury of the lens capsule heals, resulting in a stationary focal cortical cataract (AAO, 2011).

Intralenticular Foreign Bodies

In rare instances, a small foreign body can perforate the cornea and the anterior lens capsule and become lodged within the lens. If the foreign body is not composed of a ferric or cupric material and the anterior lens capsule seals the perforation site, the foreign body may be retained within the lens without significant complication. Intralenticular foreign bodies may cause cataract formation in some cases but do not always lead to lens opacification (AAO, 2011).

Radiation

Ionizing Radiation

The lens is extremely sensitive to ionizing radiation; however, as much as 20 years may pass after exposure before a cataract becomes clinically apparent. This period of latency is related to the dose of radiation and to the patient's age; younger patients are more susceptible because they have more actively growing lens cells. Ionizing radiation in the x-ray range (0.001–10.0 nm wavelength) can cause cataracts in some individuals in doses as low as 2 Gy in one fraction. (A routine chest x-ray equals 0.01 Gy exposure to the thorax.) The first clinical signs of radiation-induced cataract are often punctate opacities within the posterior capsule and feathery anterior subcapsular opacities that radiate toward the equator of the lens. These opacities may progress to complete opacification of the lens (AAO, 2011).

Infrared Radiation (glassblowers' cataract)

Exposure of the eye to infrared radiation and intense heat over time can cause the outer layers of the anterior lens capsule to peel off as a single layer. Such true exfoliation of the lens capsule, in which the exfoliated outer lamella tends to scroll up on itself, is rarely seen today. Cortical cataract may be associated (AAO, 2011).

Ultraviolet Radiation

Experimental evidence suggests that the lens is susceptible to damage from ultraviolet (UV) radiation. Epidemiologic evidence indicates that long-term exposure to sunlight is associated with increased risk of cortical cataracts. Although sunlight exposure accounts for only about 10% of the total risk of cortical cataract in the general population in temperate climates, this risk is avoidable. Since exposure to UV radiation can produce other morbidity, clinicians should encourage their patients to avoid excessive sunlight exposure. Lenses sold in the United States must conform to the American National Standards Institute requirements aimed at reducing UV transmission. Prescription corrective lenses and nonprescription sunglasses decrease UV transmission by more than 80%, and wearing a hat with a brim decreases ocular sun exposure by 30%–50% (Cruickshanks et al, 1992).

Microwave Radiation

Microwave radiation has been shown to cause cataracts in laboratory animals. Human case reports and epidemiologic studies are more controversial and less conclusive than experimental studies. Cataracts caused by microwave radiation are likely to be anterior and/or posterior subcapsular opacities (Lipman et al, 1988).

Chemical Injuries

Alkali injuries to the ocular surface often result in cataract, in addition to damaging the cornea, conjunctiva, and iris. Alkali compounds penetrate the eye readily, causing an increase in aqueous pH and a decrease in the level of aqueous glucose and ascorbate. Cortical cataract formation may occur acutely or as a delayed effect of chemical injury. Because acid tends to penetrate the eye less easily than does alkali, acid injuries are less likely to result in cataract formation (AAO, 2011).

Metallosis

Siderosis Bulbi

Iron intraocular foreign bodies can result in siderosis bulbi, a condition characterized by deposition of iron molecules in the trabecular meshwork, lens epithelium, iris, and retina. The epithelium and cortical fibers of the affected lens at first show a yellowish tinge, followed later by a rusty brown discoloration. Lens involvement occurs more rapidly if the retained foreign body is embedded close to the lens. Later manifestations of siderosis bulbi are complete cortical cataract formation and retinal dysfunction (AAO, 2011).

Chalcosis

Chalcosis occurs when an intraocular copper-containing foreign body deposits copper in the Descemet membrane, anterior lens capsule, or other intraocular basement membranes. A resulting "sunflower" cataract is a petal-shaped deposition of yellow or brown pigment in the lens capsule that radiates from the anterior axial pole of the lens to the equator. Usually, this cataract causes no significant loss of vision. However, intraocular foreign bodies containing almost pure copper (more than 90%) can cause a severe inflammatory reaction and intraocular necrosis (AAO, 2011).

Electrical Injury

Electrical shock can cause protein coagulation and cataract formation. Lens manifestations are more likely when the transmission of current involves the patient's head. Initially, lens vacuoles appear in the anterior midperiphery of the lens, followed by linear opacities in the anterior subcapsular cortex. A cataract induced by an electrical injury may regress, remain stationary, or mature to complete cataract over months or years (Portellos et al, 1996).

2.3. Drug-Induced Lens Changes

Corticosteroids

Long-term use of corticosteroids may cause PSCs. The incidence of corticosteroid-induced PSCs is related to dose and duration of treatment. Cataract formation has been reported following administration of corticosteroids by several routes: systemic, topical, subconjunctival, and inhaled. The increasing use of high-dose intraocular steroids to treat retinal neovascularization and inflammation has resulted in a substantial rise in the incidence of PSCs and of steroid-induced ocular hypertension. Coincidentally, the patients who are susceptible to steroid-induced increases in intraocular pressure (IOP) are frequently those who develop PSCs after intravitreal injection of triamcinolone acetonide. The advent of slow-release steroid repositories such as fluocinolone acetonide 0.59 mg and dexamethasone intravitreal implant 0.7 mg has not altered the IOP-elevating and PSC-producing effects of these medications on the eye (Urban and Cotlier, 1986;

van den Brûle et al, 1998; Fraunfelder and Fraunfelder, 2001; Gillies and al, 2005; Jaffe et al, 2006; Kiernan and Mieler, 2009).

Histologically and clinically, PSC formation occurring subsequent to corticosteroid use cannot be distinguished from senescent PSC formation. Some steroid-induced PSCs in children may resolve with cessation of the drug (AAO, 2011).

Phenothiazines

Phenothiazines, a major group of psychotropic medications, can cause pigmented deposits in the anterior lens epithelium in an axial configuration. The occurrence of these deposits appears to be dependent on both drug dose and treatment duration. In addition, they are more likely to be seen with the use of some phenothiazines, notably chlorpromazine and thioridazine, than with others. The visual changes associated with phenothiazine use are generally insignificant (AAO, 2011).

Miotics

The use of anticholinesterases can cause cataracts. The incidence of cataracts has been reported as high as 20% in patients after 55 months of pilocarpine use and 60% in patients after echothiophate iodide use. Usually, this type of cataract first appears as small vacuoles within and posterior to the anterior lens capsule and epithelium. These vacuoles are best appreciated on retroillumination. The cataract may progress to posterior cortical and nuclear lens changes. Cataract formation is more likely in patients receiving anticholinesterase therapy over a long period and in those receiving more frequent dosing. Although visually significant cataracts are common in elderly patients using topical anticholinesterases, progressive cataract formation has not been reported in children given echothiophate for the treatment of accommodative esotropia. The use of these medications has declined with the advent of other classes of medications for the treatment of glaucoma, and indirect-acting anticholinesterase agents are irritating, cataractogenic, and difficult to obtain.

Amiodarone

The use of amiodarone, an antiarrhythmia medication, has been reported to cause stellate pigment deposition in the anterior cortical axis. Only very rarely is this condition visually significant. Amiodarone is also deposited in the corneal epithelium and can cause a rare optic neuropathy.

Statins

Studies in dogs showed that some 3-hydroxy-3-methylglutaryl coenzyme A (HMG-CoA) reductase inhibitors (statins) are associated with cataract when given in excessive doses. Long-term use of statins in humans has been shown not to be associated with an increased cataract risk; moreover, a longitudinal study reported a 50% reduction in the 5-year incidence of nuclear cataracts in patients treated with statins. However, concomitant use of simvastatin and erythromycin, which increases circulating statin levels, may be associated with approximately a twofold increased risk of cataract (Schlienger et al, 2001; Klein et al, 2006).

Tamoxifen

In a recent study, the association previously suggested between cataract development and tamoxifen use was not substantiated. Research on and discussion of this subject continue (Bradbury and al, 2004).

2.4. Congenital Cataracts

Congenital cataracts may be unilateral or bilateral. They can be classified by morphology, presumed or defined genetic etiology, presence of specific metabolic disorders, or associated ocular anomalies or systemic findings. In general, approximately one-third of congenital cataracts are a component of a more extensive syndrome or disease (eg, cataract resulting from congenital rubella syndrome), one-third occur as an isolated inherited trait, and one-third result from undetermined causes. Metabolic diseases tend to be more commonly associated with bilateral cataracts. Congenital cataracts are genetically heterogeneous (Scott et al, 1994). It is known that different mutations in different genes can cause similar cataract patterns, while the highly variable cataract morphologies within some families suggest that the same mutation in a single gene can lead to different phenotypes (Héon et al, 1999; Gill et al, 2000).

Congenital cataracts occur in a variety of morphologic configurations, including lamellar, polar, sutural, coronary, cerulean, nuclear, capsular, cerulean, pulverulent, coralliform, wedge-shaped, polymorphic, other minor subtypes, complete, and membranous (Reddy et al, 2004; AAO, 2011).

Morphological Types (AAO, 2011)

Lamellar

Of the congenital cataracts, lamellar, or zonular, cataracts are the most common type. They are characteristically bilateral and symmetric, and their effect on visual acuity varies with the size and density of the opacity. Lamellar cataracts may be inherited as an autosomal dominant trait. In some cases, they may occur as a result of a transient toxic influence during embryonic lens development. The earlier this toxic influence occurs, the smaller and deeper is the resulting lamellar cataract.

Lamellar cataracts are opacifications of specific layers or zones of the lens. Clinically, the cataract is visible as an opacified layer that surrounds a clearer center and is itself surrounded by a layer of clear cortex. Viewed from the front, the lamellar cataract has a disc-shaped configuration. Often, additional arcuate opacities within the cortex straddle the equator of the lamellar cataract; these horseshoe-shaped opacities are called riders.

Polar

Polar cataracts are lens opacities that involve the subcapsular cortex and capsule of the anterior or posterior pole of the lens. Anterior polar cataracts are usually small, bilateral, symmetric, nonprogressive opacities that do not impair vision. They may be pyramidal and project into the anterior chamber. They are frequently inherited in an autosomal dominant pattern. Anterior polar cataracts are sometimes seen in association with other ocular abnormalities, including microphthalmos, persistent pupillary membrane, Peters anomaly, aniridia and anterior lenticonus. They do not require treatment but often cause anisometropia (AAO, 2011).

Posterior polar cataracts generally produce more visual impairment than do anterior polar cataracts because they tend to be larger and are positioned closer to the nodal point of the eye. Capsular fragility has been reported. Posterior polar cataracts are usually stable but occasionally progress. They may be familial or sporadic. Familial posterior polar cataracts are usually bilateral and inherited in an autosomal dominant pattern. Sporadic posterior polar cataracts are often unilateral and may be associated with remnants of the tunica vasculosa lentis or with an abnormality of the posterior capsule such as lenticonus or lentiglobus orpersistent hyperplastic primary vitreous (AAO, 2011).

Sutural

The sutural, or stellate, cataract is an opacification of the Y-sutures (anterior or posterior) of the fetal nucleus. It usually does not impair vision. These opacities often have branches or knobs projecting from them. Sutural cataracts are bilateral and symmetric and are frequently inherited in an autosomal dominant pattern.

Coronary

Coronary cataracts are so named because they consist of a group of club-shaped cortical opacities that are arranged around the equator of the lens like a crown, or corona. They cannot be seen unless the pupil is dilated, and they usually do not affect visual acuity. Coronary cataracts are often inherited in an autosomal dominant pattern.

Cerulean

Cerulean cataracts are small bluish opacities located in the lens cortex; hence, they are also known as blue-dot cataracts. They are nonprogressive and usually do not cause visual symptoms.

Nuclear

Congenital nuclear cataracts are opacities of the embryonic nucleus alone or of both embryonic and fetal nuclei. They are usually bilateral, with a wide spectrum of severity. Lens opacification may involve the complete nucleus or be limited to discrete layers within the nucleus. Eyes with congenital nuclear cataracts tend to be microphthalmic, and they are at increased risk of developing aphakic glaucoma.

Capsular

Capsular cataracts are small opacifications of the lens epithelium and anterior lens capsule that spare the cortex. They are differentiated from anterior polar cataracts by their protrusion into the anterior chamber. Capsular cataracts generally do not adversely affect vision.

Complete

With complete, or total, cataract, all of the lens fibers are opacified. The red reflex is completely obscured, and the retina cannot be seen with either direct or indirect ophthalmoscopy. Some cataracts may be subtotal at birth and progress rapidly to become complete cataracts. Complete cataracts may be unilateral or bilateral, and they produce profound visual impairment.

Membranous

Membranous cataracts occur when lens proteins are resorbed from either an intact or a traumatized lens, allowing the anterior and posterior lens capsules to fuse into a dense white membrane. The resulting opacity and lens distortion generally cause significant visual disability.

Congenital Anomalies and Abnormalities

Congenital Aphakia

The lens is absent in congenital aphakia, a very rare anomaly. Two forms of congenital aphakia have been described. In primary aphakia, the lens placode fails to form from the surface ectoderm in the developing embryo. In secondary aphakia, the more common type, the developing lens is spontaneously absorbed. Both forms of aphakia are usually associated with other malformations of the eye.

Lenticonus and Lentiglobus

Lenticonus is a localized, cone-shaped deformation of the anterior or posterior lens surface. Posterior lenticonus is more common than anterior lenticonus and is usually unilateral and axial in location. Anterior lenticonus is often bilateral and may be associated with Alport syndrome.

In lentiglobus, the localized deformation of the lens surface is spherical. Posterior lentiglobus is more common than anterior lentiglobus and is often associated with posterior pole opacities that vary in density.

Retinoscopy through the center of the lens reveals a distorted and myopic reflex in both lenticonus and lentiglobus. These deformations can also be seen in the red reflex, where, by retroillumination, they appear as an "oil droplet." The posterior bulging may progress with initial worsening of the myopia, followed by opacification of the defect. Surrounding cortical lamellae may also opacify (AAO, 2011).

Lens Coloboma

A lens coloboma is an anomaly of lens shape. Lens colobomas can be classified into 2 types: primary coloboma, a wedge-shaped defect or indentation of the lens periphery that occurs as an isolated anomaly; and secondary coloboma, a flattening or indentation of the lens periphery caused by the lack of ciliary body or zonular development. Lens colobomas are typically located inferiorly and may be associated with colobomas of the uvea. Cortical lens opacification or thickening of the lens capsule may appear adjacent to the coloboma. The zonular attachments in the region of the coloboma usually are weakened or absent.

Mittendorf Dot

Mittendorf dot is a common anomaly observed in many healthy eyes. A small, dense white spot generally located inferonasal to the posterior pole of the lens, a Mittendorf dot is a remnant of the posterior pupillary membrane of the tunica vasculosa lentis. It marks the place where the hyaloid artery came into contact with the posterior surface of the lens in utero. Sometimes a Mittendorf dot is associated with a fibrous tail or remnant of the hyaloid artery projecting into the vitreous body (AAO, 2011).

Epicapsular Star

Another very common remnant of the tunica vasculosa lentis is an epicapsular star. As its name suggests, this anomaly is a star-shaped distribution of tiny brown or golden flecks on the central anterior lens capsule. It may be unilateral or bilateral.

Peters Anomaly

Peters anomaly is part of a spectrum of disorders known as *anterior segment dysgenesis syndrome,* also referred to as neurocristopathy or mesodermal dysgenesis. Peters anomaly is characterized by a central or paracentral corneal opacity (leukoma) associated with thinning or absence of adjacent endothelium and Descemet membrane. In normal ocular development, the lens vesicle separates from the surface ectoderm (the future corneal epithelium) at about 33 days' gestation. Peters anomaly is typically linked with the absence of this separation. It is often associated with mutations in or deletion of 1 allele of the genes normally involved in anterior segment development, including the transcription factors *PAX6, PITX2,* and *FOXC1.* Patients with Peters anomaly may also display the following lens anomalies:

- adhesions between lens and cornea
- anterior cortical or polar cataract
- a misshapen lens displaced anteriorly into the pupillary space and the anterior chamber
- microspherophakia

Microspherophakia

Microspherophakia is a developmental abnormality in which the lens is small in diameter and spherical. The entire lens equator can be visualized at the slit lamp when the pupil is widely dilated. The spherical shape of the lens results in increased refractive power, which causes the eye to be highly myopic.

Faulty development of the secondary lens fibers during embryogenesis is believed to be the cause of microspherophakia. Microspherophakia is most often seen as a part of Weill-Marchesani syndrome, but it may also occur as an isolated hereditary abnormality or, occasionally, in association with Peters anomaly, Marfan syndrome, Alport syndrome, Lowe syndrome, or congenital rubella. Individuals with Weill-Marchesani syndrome commonly have small stature, short and stubby fingers, and broad hands with reduced joint mobility. Weill-Marchesani syndrome is usually inherited as an autosomal recessive trait (AAO, 2011).

The spherical lens can block the pupil, causing secondary angle-closure glaucoma. Use of miotics aggravates this condition by increasing pupillary block and allowing additional forward lens displacement. Cycloplegics are the medical treatment of choice to break an attack of angle-closure glaucoma in patients with microspherophakia, because they decrease pupillary block by tightening the zonular fibers, decreasing the anteroposterior lens diameter, and pulling the lens posteriorly. A laser iridotomy may also be useful in relieving angle closure in patients with microspherophakia (AAO, 2011).

Aniridia

Aniridia is an uncommon panocular syndrome in which the most dramatic manifestation is partial or nearly complete absence of the iris. Aniridia has been linked to the loss of 1 allele of the *PAX6* gene, a transcription factor that is important for the development and function of the cornea, lens, and retina. Associated findings include corneal pannus and epitheliopathy, glaucoma, foveal and optic nerve hypoplasia, and nystagmus. Aniridia is almost always bilateral. Two-thirds of cases are familial; one-third of cases are sporadic. Sporadic cases of aniridia are associated with a high incidence of Wilms tumor and the WAGR complex (Wilms tumor, aniridia, genitourinary malformations, and mental retardation).

Anterior and posterior polar lens opacities may be present at birth in patients with aniridia. Cortical, subcapsular, and lamellar opacities develop in 50%–85% of patients within the first 2 decades of life. The lens opacities may progress and further impair vision. Poor zonular integrity and ectopia lentis have also been reported in patients with aniridia (AAO, 2011).

Developmental Defects

Ectopia Lentis

Ectopia lentis is a displacement of the lens that may be congenital, developmental, or acquired. A subluxated lens is partially displaced from its normal position but remains in the pupillary area. A luxated, or dislocated, lens is completely displaced from the pupil, implying separation of all zonular attachments. Findings associated with lens subluxation include decreased vision, marked astigmatism, monocular diplopia, and iridodonesis (tremulous iris). Potential complications of ectopia lentis include cataract and displacement of the lens into the anterior chamber or into the vitreous. Dislocation into the anterior chamber or pupil may cause pupillary block and angle-closure glaucoma. Dislocation of the lens posteriorly into the vitreous cavity often has no adverse sequelae aside from a profound change in refractive error (AAO, 2011).

Trauma is the most common cause of acquired lens displacement. Nontraumatic ectopia lentis is commonly associated with Marfan syndrome, homocystinuria, aniridia, and congenital glaucoma. Less frequently, it appears with Ehlers-Danlos syndrome, hyperlysinemia, and sulfite oxidase deficiency. Ectopia lentis may occur as an isolated anomaly (simple ectopia lentis), usually inherited as an autosomal dominant trait. Ectopia lentis can also be associated with pupillary abnormalities in the ocular syndrome ectopia lentis et pupillae (AAO, 2011).

Marfan Syndrome

Marfan syndrome is a heritable disorder with ocular, cardiac, and skeletal manifestations. Though usually inherited as an autosomal dominant trait, the disorder appears with no family history in approximately 15% of cases. Marfan syndrome is caused by mutations in the fibrillin gene on chromosome 15. Affected individuals are tall, with arachnodactyly and chest wall deformities. Associated cardiac abnormalities include dilated aortic root and mitral valve prolapse (AAO, 2011).

From 50% to 80% of patients with Marfan syndrome exhibit ectopia lentis. The lens subluxation tends to be bilateral and symmetric (usually superior and temporal), but variations do occur. The zonular attachments commonly remain intact but become stretched and elongated. Ectopia lentis in

Marfan syndrome is probably congenital in most cases. Progression of lens subluxation is observed in some patients over time, but in many patients the lens position remains stable.

Ocular abnormalities associated with Marfan syndrome include axial myopia and an increased risk of retinal detachment. Patients with Marfan syndrome may develop pupillary block glaucoma if the lens dislocates into the pupil or anterior chamber. Open-angle glaucoma may also occur. In addition, children with lens subluxation may develop amblyopia if their refractive error shows significant asymmetry or remains uncorrected in early childhood (AAO, 2011).

Spectacle or contact lens correction of the refractive error provides satisfactory visual acuity in most cases. Pupillary dilation is sometimes helpful. The clinician may refract both the phakic and the aphakic portions of the pupil to determine the optimum visual acuity. A reading add is often necessary because the subluxated lens lacks sufficient accommodation (AAO, 2011).

In some cases, adequate visual acuity cannot be obtained with spectacle or contact lens correction, and removal of the lens may be indicated. Lens extraction—either extracapsular or intracapsular—in patients with Marfan syndrome is associated with a high rate of complications such as vitreous loss and complex retinal detachment. Improved results have been reported with lensectomy using vitrectomy instrumentation, although the long-term results are not yet known (AAO, 2011).

Homocystinuria

Homocystinuria is an autosomal recessive disorder, an inborn error of methionine metabolism. Serum levels of homocystine and methionine are elevated. Affected individuals are healthy at birth but develop seizures and osteoporosis and soon display mental disability. They are usually tall and have light-colored hair. Patients with homocystinuria are also prone to thromboembolic episodes, and surgery and general anesthesia are thought to increase the risk of thromboembolism.

Lens dislocation in homocystinuria tends to be bilateral and symmetric. The dislocation appears in infancy in approximately 30% of affected individuals, and by the age of 15 years, it appears in 80% of those affected. The lenses are usually subluxated inferiorly and nasally, but variations have been reported. Because zonular fibers of the lens are known to have a high concentration of cysteine, deficiency of cysteine is thought to disturb normal zonular development; affected fibers tend to be brittle and easily disrupted.

Studies of infants with homocystinuria treated with a low-methionine, high-cysteine diet and vitamin supplementation with the coenzyme pyridoxine (vitamin B6) have shown that this therapy holds promise in reducing the incidence of ectopia lentis (AAO, 2011).

Hyperlysinemia

Hyperlysinemia, an inborn error of metabolism of the amino acid lysine, is associated with ectopia lentis. Affected individuals also show mental disability and muscular hypotony.

Genetic Contributions to Age-Related Cataracts

Studies of identical and fraternal twins and of familial associations suggest that a large proportion of the risk of age-related cataracts is inherited. It is estimated that inheritance accounts for more than 50% of the risk of cortical cataracts. Recent studies identified mutations in the gene associated with congenital and age-related cortical cataracts, *EPHA2,* which has been mapped to 1p36. This is the first gene known to cause hereditary, nonsyndromic age-related cortical cataracts, although mutations at this locus account for only a small fraction of cortical opacities. Similarly, 35%–50% of the risk of nuclear cataracts can be traced to inheritance. Identification of the genes associated with increased risk of cortical and nuclear cataracts is important, because understanding the biochemical pathways in which they function may suggest ways to slow the progression or prevent the development of age-related cataracts in a large number of cases (Jun et al, 2009; Shields et al, 2008).

Ectopia Lentis et Pupillae

In the autosomal recessive disorder ectopia lentis et pupillae, the lens and the pupil are displaced in opposite directions. The pupil is irregular, usually slit shaped, and displaced from the normal position. The dislocated lens may bisect the pupil or may be completely luxated from the pupillary space. This disorder is usually bilateral but not symmetric. Characteristically, the iris dilates poorly. Associated ocular anomalies include severe axial myopia, retinal detachment, enlarged corneal diameter, cataract, and abnormal iris transillumination (AAO, 2011).

Persistent Fetal Vasculature

Persistent fetal vasculature (PFV), also known as *persistent hyperplastic primary vitreous (PHPV),* is a congenital, nonhereditary ocular malformation that frequently involves the lens. In 90% of patients, it is unilateral. A white, fibrous retrolental tissue is present, often in association with posterior cortical opacification. Progressive cataract formation often occurs, sometimes leading to a complete cataract. Other abnormalities associated with PFV include elongated ciliary processes, prominent radial iris vessels, and persistent hyaloid artery (AAO, 2011).

2.5. Metabolic Cataract

Diabetes Mellitus
Diabetes mellitus can affect lens clarity as well as the refractive index and accommodative amplitude of the lens. As the blood glucose level increases, so, also, does the glucose content in the aqueous humor. Acute myopic shifts may indicate undiagnosed or poorly controlled diabetes. Patients with type 1 diabetes have a decreased amplitude of accommodation compared to age-matched controls, and presbyopia may present at a younger age in patients with diabetes (AAO, 2011).

Cataract is a common cause of visual impairment in patients with diabetes. Acute diabetic cataract, or "snowflake" cataract, consists of bilateral, widespread subcapsular lens changes of abrupt onset, typically in young people with uncontrolled diabetes mellitus. Multiple gray-white subcapsular opacities that have a snowflake appearance are seen initially in the superficial anterior and posterior lens cortex. Vacuoles and clefts form in the underlying cortex. Intumescence and maturity of the cortical cataract follow shortly thereafter. Although acute diabetic cataracts are rarely encountered in clinical practice today, rapidly maturing bilateral cortical cataracts in a child or young adult should alert the clinician to the possibility of diabetes mellitus (AAO, 2011).

Diabetic patients develop age-related lens changes that are indistinguishable from nondiabetic age-related cataracts, except that these lens changes tend to occur at a younger age in patients with diabetes than in those without the disease. The increased risk or earlier onset of age-related cataracts in diabetic patients may be a result of the accumulation of sorbitol within the lens and accompanying changes in hydration, increased nonenzymatic glycosylation (glycation) of lens proteins, or greater oxidative stress from alterations in lens metabolism (Gold and Weingest, 1990; Flynn and Smiddy, 2000).

Galactosemia

Galactosemia is an inherited autosomal recessive inability to convert galactose to glucose. As a consequence of this inability, excessive galactose accumulates in body tissues, with further metabolic conversion of galactose to galactitol (dulcitol), the sugar alcohol of galactose. Galactosemia can result from defects in 1 of 3 enzymes involved in the metabolism of galactose: galactose 1-phosphate uridyltransferase (Gal-1-PUT), galactokinase, or UDPgalactose 4-epimerase. The most common and the severest form, known as classic galactosemia, is caused by a defect in Gal-1-PUT (AAO, 2011).

In classic galactosemia, symptoms of malnutrition, hepatomegaly, jaundice, and mental deficiency present within the first few weeks of life. The disease is fatal if undiagnosed and untreated. The diagnosis of classic galactosemia can be confirmed by demonstration of galactose in the urine.

Typically, the nucleus and deep cortex become increasingly opacified, causing an "oil droplet" appearance on retroillumination. If the disease remains untreated, the cataracts progress to total opacification. Treatment of galactosemia includes elimination of milk and milk products from the diet. In some cases, early cataract formation can be reversed by timely diagnosis and dietary intervention (Burke et al, 1989).

Deficiencies of the 2 other enzymes, galactokinase and epimerase, can also cause galactosemia. These deficiencies are less common, however, and cause less severe systemic abnormalities. Cataracts caused by deficiencies in these enzymes tend to present later in life than those seen in classic galactosemia.

Hypocalcemia

Cataracts may occur in association with any condition that results in hypocalcemia. Hypocalcemia may be idiopathic, or it may appear as a result of unintended destruction of the parathyroid glands during thyroid surgery. Usually bilateral, hypocalcemic (tetanic) cataracts are punctate iridescent opacities in the anterior and posterior cortex. They lie beneath the lens capsule and are usually separated from it by a zone of clear lens. These discrete opacities may remain stable or may mature into complete cortical cataracts (AAO, 2011).

Wilson Disease

Wilson disease (hepatolenticular degeneration) is an inherited autosomal recessive disorder of copper metabolism. The characteristic ocular manifestation of Wilson disease is the Kayser-Fleischer ring, a golden brown discoloration of the Descemet membrane around the periphery of the cornea. In addition, a characteristic "sunflower" cataract often develops. Reddish brown pigment (cuprous oxide) is deposited in the anterior lens capsule and subcapsular cortex in a stellate shape that resembles the petals of a sunflower. In most cases, the sunflower cataract does not produce serious visual impairment (AAO, 2011).

2.6. Other Morphological Cataracts

Myotonic Dystrophy

Myotonic dystrophy is an inherited autosomal dominant condition characterized by delayed relaxation of contracted muscles, ptosis, weakness of the facial musculature, cardiac conduction defects, and prominent frontal balding in affected male patients. Patients with this disorder typically develop polychromatic iridescent crystals in the lens cortex, with sequential PSC progressing to complete cortical opacification. These crystals are also noted unilaterally in patients without myotonic dystrophy. Ultrastructurally, polychromatic iridescent crystals are composed of whorls of plasmalemma from the lens fibers. The crystals are occasionally seen in the lens cortex of patients who do not have myotonic dystrophy; these crystals are thought to be caused by cholesterol crystal deposition in the lens (AAO, 2011).

Rubella

Maternal infection with the rubella virus, an RNA togavirus, can cause fetal damage, especially if the infection occurs during the first trimester of pregnancy. Systemic manifestations of congenital rubella infection include cardiac defects, deafness, and mental disability. Cataracts resulting from congenital rubella syndrome are characterized by pearly white nuclear opacifications. Sometimes the entire lens is opacified (complete cataract), and the cortex may liquefy. Histologically, lens-fiber nuclei are retained deep within the lens substance. Live virus particles may be recovered from the lens as late as 3 years after the patient's birth. Cataract removal may be complicated by excessive postoperative inflammation caused by release of these live virus particles. Other ocular manifestations of congenital rubella syndrome include diffuse pigmentary retinopathy, microphthalmos, glaucoma, and transient or permanent corneal clouding. Although congenital rubella syndrome may cause cataract or glaucoma, both conditions are usually not present simultaneously in the same eye (AAO, 2011).

Other intrauterine infections that may be associated with neonatal cataract are toxoplasmosis, cytomegalovirus, herpes simplex and varicella.

Systemic Syndromes

There are many syndromes associated with neonatal cataract. The most important are (Kanski, 2002):

Lowe (oculocerebrorenal syndrome) syndrome, which is a rare inborn error of amino acid metabolism which predominantly, affects boys. It is one of the few conditions in which congenital glaucoma and congenital cataract coexist. Inheritance is X-linked recessive. Systemic features include mental handicap, renal dwarfism, osteomalacia, muscvular hypotonia and frontal prominence. Congenital cataract is universal. The lens is small, thin and disc-like (microphakia), and may show posterior lentiglobus. The lens opacities mat be capsular, lamellar, nuclear or total. Mothers of affected children may also show multiple punctate lens opacities. Congenital glaucoma is present in 50% of cases.

Hallerman-Streiff-Francois syndrome: systemic features include dyscephaly with a small thin nose, hypotrichosis, dental anomalies, and postnatal growth retardation. Congenital cataract, which may be membranous, is universal. Other ocular features include blue sclera, strabismus and disc coloboma.

The following shromosomal disorders are associated with cataracts: Down syndrome (trisomy 21), Patau syndrome (trisomy 13), Edward syndrome (trisomy 18), Cri-du-chat syndrome (deletion of chromosome 5) and Turner syndrome.

Other syndromes include Nance-Horan, Rubenstein-Taybi and Marinesco-Sjögren.

Cataract Associated with Uveitis

Lens changes often occur as a result of chronic uveitis or associated corticosteroid therapy. Typically, a PSC appears; anterior lens changes may also occur. The formation of posterior synechiae is common in uveitis, often with thickening of the anterior lens capsule, which may have an associated fibrous pupillary membrane. Lens changes in cataract secondary to uveitis may progress to a mature cataract. Calcium deposits may be observed on the anterior capsule or within the lens substance (AAO, 2011).

Cortical cataract formation occurs in up to 70% of cases of Fuchs heterochromic uveitis. Because posterior synechiae do not commonly occur in this syndrome, formation of pupillary membranes is unlikely, and long-term corticosteroid therapy is not indicated. Cataract extraction in patients with Fuchs heterochromic uveitis generally has a favorable prognosis. Intraoperative anterior chamber hemorrhages have been reported in approximately 25% of cases (AAO, 2011).

Cataracts Associated with Ocular Treatments

Posterior subcapsular cataract secondary to corticosteroid treatment is discussed in the previous section. Vitrectomy is another cause of treatment-induced cataract. Transient opacities involving the posterior sutures can occur soon after vitrectomy, but these opacities usually resolve spontaneously. However, more than 60% and up to 95% of patients who undergo vitrectomy during surgical treatment of a variety of retinal problems develop nuclear cataracts within 2 years of the surgery. Postvitrectomy cataracts are less common in patients younger than 50 years. The formation of nuclear cataracts after vitrectomy is associated with increases in oxygen tension in the vitreous intraoperatively and postoperatively. (See Chapter 2 for a discussion of oxygen tension in the lens.) Retinal surgery performed without vitrectomy is not associated with increased lens opacification. In this regard, age-related degeneration of the vitreous body has also been associated with increased risk of nuclear opacification (AAO, 2011).

Cataracts and Hyperbaric Oxygen Therapy

Lens changes may also occur after hyperbaric oxygen therapy. Several studies found a myopic shift during the course of several weeks of hyperbaric oxygen therapy for different conditions. Since no change in axial length or corneal curvature was detected, the refractive change was presumed to be due to increased nuclear sclerosis. In most cases, the myopic shift resolved after cessation of therapy. In patients exposed to hyperbaric oxygen at least 150 times during a 1-year period, nearly 50% of patients with previously clear lenses developed frank nuclear cataracts, consistent with the increase in oxygenation in the vitreous. An increase in nuclear light scatter was shown in most of the other patients in this treatment group when they were compared with older, sicker patients who were in the same clinic but not eligible for hyperbaric oxygen therapy (Palmquist et al, 1984).

Exfoliation Syndrome

Exfoliation syndrome (pseudoexfoliation) is a systemic disease in which a matrix of fibrotic material is deposited in many bodily organs. In the eye, a basement membrane–like fibrillogranular white material is deposited on the lens, cornea, iris, anterior hyaloid face, ciliary processes, zonular fibers, and trabecular meshwork. These deposits, believed to comprise elastic microfibrils, appear as grayish white flecks that are prominent at the pupillary margin and on the lens capsule. Associated with this condition are atrophy of the iris at the pupillary margin, deposition of pigment on the anterior surface of the iris, poorly dilating pupil, increased pigmentation of the trabecular meshwork, capsular fragility, zonular weakness, and open-angle glaucoma. Exfoliation syndrome is a unilateral or bilateral disorder that becomes more apparent with increasing age.

Increased oxidative stress caused by abnormalities in transforming growth factor β (TGF-β) contributes to the formation of cataracts. Patients with this syndrome may also experience weakness of the zonular fibers and spontaneous lens subluxation and phacodonesis. Poor zonular integrity may affect cataract surgery technique and intraocular lens implantation. The exfoliative material may be elaborated even after the crystalline lens is removed (Schötzer-Schrehardt and Naumann, 2006; Zenkel et al, 2010).

Cataract and Atopic Dermatitis

Atopic dermatitis is a chronic, erythematous dermatitis, accompanied by itching and often seen in conjunction with increased levels of immunoglobulin E (IgE) and a history of multiple allergies or asthma. Cataract formation has been reported in up to 25% of patients with atopic dermatitis. The cataracts are usually bilateral, and onset occurs in the second to third decade of life. Typically, these cataracts are anterior subcapsular opacities in the pupillary area that resemble shieldlike plaques (Mannis et al, 1996).

Phacoantigenic Uveitis

In the normal eye, minute amounts of lens proteins leak out through the lens capsule. The eye appears to have immunologic tolerance to these small amounts of lens antigens. However, the release of a large amount of lens protein into the anterior chamber disrupts this immunologic tolerance and may trigger a severe inflammatory reaction. Phacoantigenic uveitis, sometimes referred to as phacoanaphylactic uveitis, is an immune-mediated granulomatous inflammation initiated by lens proteins released through a ruptured lens capsule. This condition usually occurs following traumatic rupture of the lens capsule or following cataract surgery when cortical material is retained within the eye. Onset occurs days to weeks after the injury or surgery.

The disease is characterized by a red, painful eye with injection, chemosis, and anterior chamber inflammation with cells, flare, and keratic precipitates. Occasionally, glaucoma secondary to blockage of the trabecular meshwork and formation of synechiae may occur. Late complications include cyclitic membrane, hypotony, and phthisis bulbi. In rare instances, phacoantigenic uveitis can give rise to an inflammatory reaction in the fellow eye. Histologic examination shows a zonal granulomatous inflammation surrounding a breach of the lens capsule. Lens extraction is the definitive therapy for the condition (AAO, 2011).

Lens-Induced Glaucoma

Phacolytic Glaucoma

Phacolytic glaucoma is a complication of a mature or hypermature cataract. Denatured, liquefied high-molecular-mass lens proteins leak through an intact but permeable lens capsule. An immune response is not elicited; rather, macrophages ingest these lens proteins. The trabecular meshwork can become clogged with both the lens proteins and the engorged macrophages. The usual clinical presentation of phacolytic glaucoma consists of abrupt onset of pain and redness in a cataractous eye that has had poor vision for some time. The cornea may be edematous, and significant flare reaction occurs in the anterior chamber. White flocculent material appears in the anterior chamber and often adheres to the lens capsule as well. IOP is markedly elevated; and the anterior chamber angle is open, although the same material may be seen in the trabecular meshwork. Initial treatment of phacolytic glaucoma consists of controlling IOP with antiglaucoma medications and managing inflammation with topical corticosteroids. Surgical removal of the lens is the definitive treatment (AAO, 2011).

Lens Particle Glaucoma

Following a penetrating lens injury or surgical procedure (ie, extracapsular cataract extraction or phacoemulsification with retained cortical material; or, in rare instances, Nd:YAG laser capsulotomy), particles of lens cortex may migrate into the anterior chamber, where they obstruct aqueous outflow through the trabecular meshwork. In most instances, the onset of glaucoma is delayed by days or weeks after the surgical event or lens injury. Gonioscopy shows that the angle is open, and cortical material can often be seen deposited along the trabecular meshwork. Medical therapy to lower IOP and to reduce intraocular inflammation is indicated. If the IOP and inflammation do not respond quickly to this treatment, surgical removal of the retained lens material may be required (Richter and Epstein, 1996).

Phacomorphic Glaucoma

An intumescent cataractous lens can cause pupillary block and induce secondary angle-closure glaucoma, or it can physically push the iris forward and thus cause shallowing of the anterior chamber. Typically, the patient presents with a red, painful eye and a history of decreased vision as a result of cataract formation prior to the acute event. The cornea may be edematous, and gonioscopy reveals a closed anterior chamber angle. Initial management includes medical treatment to lower the IOP. The condition responds to laser iridotomy, but definitive treatment consists of cataract extraction (Liebman and Ritch, 1996).

Glaukomflecken

Glaukomflecken are gray-white epithelial and anterior cortical lens opacities that occur following an episode of markedly elevated IOP, as in acute angle-closure glaucoma. Histologically, glaukomflecken are composed of necrotic lens epithelial cells and degenerated subepithelial cortex (AAO, 2011).

Ischemia

Ischemic ocular conditions, such as pulseless disease (Takayasu arteritis), thromboangiitis obliterans (Buerger disease), and anterior segment necrosis, can cause PSC. The cataract may progress rapidly to total opacification of the lens (AAO, 2011).

Cataracts Associated with Degenerative Ocular Disorders

Cataracts can occur secondary to many degenerative ocular diseases, such as retinitis pigmentosa, essential iris atrophy, chronic hypotony, and absolute glaucoma. These secondary cataracts usually begin as PSCs and may progress to total lens opacification. The mechanisms responsible for cataractogenesis in degenerative ocular disorders are not well understood.

3. Different Types of Cataracts

Cataracts may be partial or complete, stationary or progressive, or hard or soft.There are several different types of cataracts, each defined by their location on the lens: nuclear, cortical (spoke-like or oil droplet), subcapsular (anterior and posterior), and mixed. Each type has its own anatomical location, pathology, and risk factors for development. The main (primary) types of age-related cataracts are nuclear sclerosis, cortical, and posterior subcapsular. As a person ages, any one type, or a combination of any of these three types can develop over time (Figure 1 and 2). A mature cataract is one in which all of the lens protein is opaque while the immature cataract has some transparent protein. In the hypermature cataract, also known as Morgagnian cataract the lens proteins have become liquid. Congenital cataract, has a different classification and includes lamellar, polar, sutural, coronary, cerulean, nuclear, capsular, complete, and membranous cataract (Figure 3) (Spencer and Andelman, 1965; Greiner and Chylack, 1979).

Several systems are available to classify and grade lens opacities (Vivino et al, 1993; Magno et al, 1994; Chylack et al, 1993; Taylor and West, 1989; Klein et al, 1990). Cataracts can be classified by using Lens Opacities Classification System III. In this system, cataract is classified based on type as nuclear, cortical, or posterior. The cataracts are further classified based on severity on a scale from 1 to 5. Research has demonstrated that the LOCS III system is highly reproducible (Yanoff and Duker, 2009).

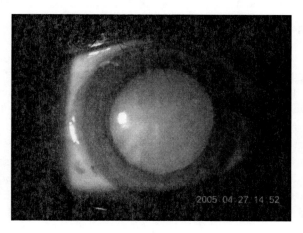

Figure 1. Hypermature cataract (age related cataract).

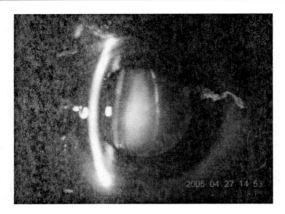

Figure 2. Mixed cataract (nuclear and subcapsular posterior).

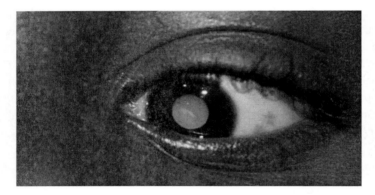

Figure 3. Congenital cataract (total).

Nuclear cataracts consist of a central opacification or coloration that interferes with visual function. Nuclear cataracts are found in the center, or nucleus of the lens and are the commonest types of cataracts.There are different types of nuclear cataracts, accompanied by either brunescence, opalescence, or both (Ventura et al, 1987). Nuclear cataracts tend to progress slowly and affect distance vision more than near vision. In advanced cases, the lens becomes brown and opaque. This type of cataract can present with a shift to nearsightedness and causes problems with distance vision while reading is less affected (Bollinger and Langston, 2008). Cortical cataracts can be central or peripheral and sometimes are best appreciated by retroillumination or retinoscopy. Cataracts affect the edges of the lens. A cortical cataract begins as whitish, wedge-shaped opacities or streaks on the outer edge of the lens cortex. As it slowly progresses, the streaks extend to the center and interfere with light passing through the center of the lens. Problems with glare are common for people with this type of cataract.A cortical cataract is characterized by white, wedge-like opacities that start in the periphery of the lens and work their way to the center in a spoke-like fashion. This type of cataract occurs in the lens cortex, which is the part of the lens that surrounds the central nucleus. Patients with this type of cataract commonly complain of glare. When the entire cortex becomes white and opaque, the cataract is referred to as a mature cortical cataract. Cortical cataracts are due to opacification of the lens cortex (outer layer). They occur when changes in the water content of the periphery of the lens causes fissuring. When these cataracts are viewed through an ophthalmoscope or other magnification system, the appearance is similar to white spokes of a wheel pointing inwards. Symptoms often include problems with glare and light catter at night (Bollinger and Langston, 2008).

Posterior subcapsular (PSC) cataracts *affect the back of the lens (posterior subcapsular cataracts)*. A posterior subcapsular cataract starts as a small, opaque area that usually forms near the back of the lens, right in the path of light on its way to the retina. A subcapsular cataract often interferes with your reading vision, reduces your vision in bright light. It causes glare or halos around lights at night and can cause significant visual impairment if they affect the axial region of the lens. Posterior subcapsular cataracts are found more often in younger patients than are nuclear or cortical cataracts. Patients often have glare and poor vision with bright lighting, and their near vision is typically more affected than distance vision. Two population-based studies found that of the three types, PSC cataracts are associated with the greatest rate of cataract surgery (Klein et al, 1997; Panchapakesan et al, 2003). In an older population (mean age 79 years) undergoing cataract surgery, however, nuclear cataracts were most frequently encountered (Lewis et al, 2004). Posterior subcapsular cataracts are cloudy at back of the lens adjacent to the capsule (or bag) in which the lens sits. Because light becomes more focused toward the back of the lens, they can cause disproportionate symptoms for their size.

Anterior Subcapsular Cataract Lies Directely under the Lens Capsule

Congenital Cataract

Congenital cataracts refer to cataracts that are present from birth, or are developed in early childhood, and may include nuclear, cortical, subcapsular or total cataracts. Congenital cataracts may be linked to an infection contracted by the mother during pregnancy, or to a genetic condition such as Fabry's disease, Alport syndrome, or galactosemia.

4. Risk Factors for Cataracts

Identification and awareness of risk factors for cataract could have an important benefit. Estimates are that if cataract onset could be delayed by 10 years, the number of cataract surgeries could be reduced annually by 45% (West 1995). Risk factors include:

4.1. Age

Many factors are associated with age-related cataract. Age is an important risk factor for senile cataract. As a person ages, the chance of developing a senile cataract increases. In the Framingham Eye Study from 1973-1975, the number of total and new cases of senile cataract rose dramatically from 23.0 cases per 100,000 and 3.5 cases per 100,000, respectively, in persons aged 45-64 years to 492.2 cases per 100,000 and 40.8 cases per 100,000 in persons aged 85 years and older.

The link between older age and cataract has been well reported. Older age was found to be a risk factor for the development of nuclear, cortical, and mixed lens opacities in the Longitudinal Los Angeles Latino Eye Study (LALES) investigation (Richter et al, 2012). Both the Barbados Eye Study and the Age-Related Eye Disease Study (AREDS) found age to be a significant risk factor for incident nuclear, cortical, and posterior subcapsular lens opacities (Leske et al,2002; Hennis et al, 2004; Chang et al, 2011).

Nuclear cataracts occur as the result of changes to crystallins in the lens nucleus, and oxidation of proteins is thought to play an especially important role in this process (Truscott, 2005; Beebe et al, 2010; Takahashi et al, 2004; Zhang et al, 2012; Ates et al, 2010). Some of these lens nucleus changes have been linked to aging and are thought to contribute to hardening of the lens even before cataract formation (Beebe et al, 2010; Heys et al, 2007; Richter et al, 2012). The strong epidemiologic link between older age and nuclear cataract formation (Leske et al, 2002; Chang et al, 2011; Leske et al, 1998; Richter et al, 2012) may be the result of these age-related changes of progressive hardening and then opacification of the lens nucleus. It is possible that the cumulative exposure to such oxidative factors with older age may promote these lens protein changes and thus play a role in nuclear lens opacity formation with older age (Richter et al, 2012).

The cumulative effect of environmental factors (UV light, x-irradiation, toxins, metals, steroids, drugs, and diseases including diabetes) plays also a role. Gene expression changes result in altered enzyme, growth factor, and other protein levels. Protein modification, oxidation, conformational changes, aggregation and phase separation, formation of the nuclear barrier, increased proteolysis, defective calcium metabolism, and defense mechanisms are also important factors. Compromised ion transport leads to osmotic imbalances and intercellular vacuolation. Abnormal cellular proliferation and differentiation also produces opacities (Taylor, 2002).

Increasing age is the greatest risk factor for cataract due to cumulative exposure to risk factors together with an age-related decline in antioxidants and antioxidant enzymes (Taylor, 2002). Increasing age is also associated with an increased incidence of diseases such as diabetes (Ederer et al, 1981). The chronic cumulative effect of taking medications (such as steroids) that may cause cataracts increases the risk of developing cataracts in older people (Jobling and Augusteyn, 2002).

4.2. Gender

In the United States, women have a significantly higher age-adjusted prevalence of cataract, with 58% of cataract cases (Congdon et al, 2004). Women have a higher risk for most types of cataracts (Delcourt 2000), although evidence suggests estrogen may protect against cataract formation. The anti-estrogen drug tamoxifen (used to block estrogen receptors) increases risk of cataract when taken long-term (Cumming 1997). Female gender was found to be a risk factor for the development of posterior subcapsular opacities (Richter et al, 2012). Female gender was also an independent risk factor for prevalent mixed-type lens opacities (Richter et al, 2012). The Barbados Eye Study suggested that female gender increased the risk for incident nuclear and cortical lens opacities; the Pathologies Oculaires Liées à l'Age study demonstrated an association between female gender and prevalent cortical lens opacities and having obtained cataract surgery (Leske et al, 2002; Hennis et al, 2004; Delcourt, 2000). AREDS reported recently an increased risk of cortical cataract in females but a decreased risk of PSC, which counters findings of Chang and associates (Chang et al, 2011). Association beteween female gender and cataract may be related to differing genetic or environmental factors (Richter et al, 2012).

4.3. Education Status and Socioeconomic Factors

Risk for cataract is greater among individuals with lower socioeconomic status or educational level. This could be attributed to increased exposure to conditions inducing cataract development (eg, nutritional deficiencies from poor diet, increased exposure to disease, and poor general health) (West 1995). A higher level of education is associated with a lower risk of age-related cataract; however, this may be related to other factors such as smoking, alcohol intake, and increased sun exposure in people with less education.

4.4. Exposure to Excessive Sunlight

Geographical areas with more hours of sunlight have a greater prevalence of cataract, showing an association between ultraviolet B irradiation and cataract formation (Heck, 2004). Cataract is a multifactorial disease which is associated with many environmental (McCarty and Taylor, 2002) and genetic variations (McCarty and Taylor, 2001; Hejtmancik and Kantorow, 2004; Shiels and Hejtmancik, 2007). Epidemiologic studies have shown that cataract is associated with environmental factors such as exposure to sunlight and ultraviolet B light (McCarty and Taylor, 2002). Oxidative stress as a result of increased generation of reactive oxygen species and free radicals in the lens has been considered one of the main causes of senile cataract (Ottonello et al, 2000; Vinson, 2006). The toxic effects of oxidative stress during cataractogenesis can be alleviated by cellular defense mechanisms.

There is much evidence that UV-B light has an effect on cataractogenesis, presumably on the basis of increased oxidative damage. Aging eyes are more susceptible to UV damage because the level of free UV filters decreases with age and breakdown products of the filters can also act as photosensitizers, which promote the production of reactive oxygen species and oxidation of proteins. The risk of cortical and nuclear cataract has been shown to be highest among those with high sun exposure at younger ages. Exposure later in life resulted in weaker associations. Wearing sunglasses, particularly during the early years, affords some protective effect (Neale et al, 2003). Unfortunately, the proportion of risk attributable to sunlight exposure is small (McCarty et al,

1999), and cortical cataracts are less debilitating than nuclear or posterior subcapsular cataracts.

4.5. Exposure to Radiation

Exposure to X-rays or gamma radiation is a risk factor for cortical and posterior subcapsular cataracts in humans. Radiologists routinely minimize exposing the lens to ionizing radiation; if not possible, however, cataracts frequently develop and require surgical treatment (Worgul et al, 1976).

Ultraviolet light, specifically UV-B, has been shown to cause cataract and there is some evidence that sunglasses worn at an early age can slow its development in later life (Sliney, 1994). Most UV light from the sun is filtered out by the atmosphere but airline pilots often have high rates of cataract because of the increased levels of UV radiation in the upper atmosphere (Rafnssen et al, 2005). It is hypothesised that depletion of the ozone layer and a consequent increase in levels of UV light on the ground may increase future rates of cataracts (Dobson, 2005) It has also been recognized, from experimental animal studies and epidemiological studies in humans, that microwaves can cause cataract. The mechanism is unclear but may include changes in heat sensitive enzymes that normally protect cell proteins in the lens. Another mechanism that has been advanced is direct damage to the lens from pressure waves induced in the aqueous humor. Cataracts have also been associated with ionizing radiation such as X-rays. In addition to the mechanisms already mentioned, the addition of damage to the DNA of the lens cells has been considered (Lipman et al, 1988). Finally, electric and heat injuries denature and whiten the lens itself as a result of direct protein coagulation (Yanoff and Duker, 2009). This is the same process through which the clear albumin of an egg becomes white and opaque after cooking. These types of cataract are often seen in glass blowers and furnace workers.

Animal and retrospective studies have shown that exposure to high levels of x-rays and whole body irradiation causes cataracts.

4.6. Nutrition

A diet lacking a high intake of antioxidants (particularly vitamins A, C, and E) fails to protect the lens from cataract formation (Sarma 1994; Waagbo 2003).

Although nutritional deficiencies have been demonstrated to cause cataracts in animal models, this etiology has been difficult to confirm in humans. Numerous population-based studies have found that lower socioeconomic status, lower education level, and poorer overall nutrition are associated with increased prevalence of age-related cataracts. The identification of specific dietary deficiencies that lead to cataract formation and of supplements that protect against it has been more difficult. Some studies have suggested that taking multivitamin supplements, vitamin A, vitamin C, vitamin E, niacin, thiamine, riboflavin, beta carotene, or increased protein may have a protective effect on cataract development. Other studies have found that vitamins C and E have little or no effect on cataract development. Most recently, the Age-Related Eye Disease Study (AREDS) showed that, over 7 years, increased intake of vitamins C and E and beta carotene did not decrease the development or progression of cataract. Use of the multivitamin supplement offered to all AREDS participants was moderately protective against the development of nuclear opacities (AAO, 2011).

Lutein and zeaxanthin are the only carotenoids found in human lenses, and recent studies have shown a moderate decrease in cataract risk with the increased frequency of intake of food high in lutein (eg, spinach, kale, and broccoli). Eating cooked spinach more than twice a week decreased the risk of cataract. This decreased risk was unrelated to a healthful lifestyle. In contrast to the effects of such dietary supplements, severe episodes of diarrhea associated with severe dehydration may be linked to an increased risk of cataract formation (AAO, 2011).

4.7. Smoking and Alcohol

Smoking as an independent risk factor for the development of nuclear lens opacities, has been well demonstrated by the Blue Mountains Eye Study, the Beaver Dam Eye Study, and the Longitudinal Study of Cataract and the Los Angeles Latino Eye Study (Leske et al, 1998; Klein et al, 2003; Tan et al, 2008; Richter et al, 2012). Even exposure to indoor cooking smoke has been linked to nuclear cataract (Pokhrel et al, 2005). Smoking causes a threefold increase in the risk of developing nuclear cataracts (Klein, 2003; Nirmalan, 2004). A dose–response relationship between the amount of smoking exposure and the risk for nuclear lens opacities has also been well documented (West et al, 1989; Christen et al, 1992; Hiller et al, 1997; Tan et al, 2008). In contrast,

AREDS reported that smoking was associated with incident cortical lens opacities and cataract surgery, but no association was reported with nuclear opacities (Chang et al, 2011). Mechanisms behind smoking as a potential etiologic agent for nuclear sclerosis most likely involve oxidative damage of the lens, supported by the findings of reduced antioxidant levels in smokers; increased reactive advanced glycation end products in smokers, both in the lenses and systemically; and the direct toxicity of heavy metals from cigarette smoke to the lens (Ramakrishnan et al, 1995; Howard et al, 1998; Banerjee et al, 1998; Nicholl et al, 1998; Cekic et al, 1998; Boscia et al, 2000). Some basic science studies have suggested a particularly important role for oxidative damage in nuclear opacity development (Truscott, 2005; Simpanya et al, 2005; Beebe et al, 2010), and this is supported by the epidemiologic data demonstrating the specific relationship between smoking and nuclear opacity development.

There is limited evidence of an association between smoking and posterior subcapsular cataract, and little or no association with cortical cataract. Smokers also have a higher prevalence of other health-threatening habits such as poor diet and high alcohol consumption, which are risk factors for cataract. Smoking causes a reduction in endogenous antioxidants and tobacco smoke contains heavy metals such as cadmium, lead, and copper, which accumulate in the lens and cause toxicity (Kelly et al, 2005).

There is conflicting evidence over the effect of alcohol. Some surveys have shown a link but others that have followed patients over time have not (Wang et al, 2008). Chronic alcoholism was associated with a significantly increased risk of cataract in one study (Hiratsuka and Li, 2001). Risk for all cataract types increase with heavy alcohol consumption (Delcourt 2000). Consumption of alcohol, particularly hard liquor and wine, was associated with nuclear opacities. Wine drinking was inversely related to cortical opacity (Morris et al, 2004). Some studies have not shown an association between alcohol consumption and cataracts (Klein et al, 2003).

4.8. Diabetes

Diabetics are more likely to develop cortical opacities or require cataract surgery (Klein et al, 2002).The relationship of diabetes and poor diabetic control with incidence of various lens opacities has been well documented in large epidemiologic studies, including the Barbados Eye Study, Beaver Dam Eye Study, Pathologies Oculaires Liées à l'Age Study, AREDS and the Los

Angeles Latino Eye Study (Klein et al, 1995; Leske et al, 1999; Delcourt et al, 2000; Chang et al,2011; Richter et al, 2012). The role of the polyol pathway is evoqued in the chronology of events, whereby aldose reductase catalyzes the reduction of glucose to sorbitol, in the initiation of diabetic lens changes (Varma, 1980). This leads to an osmotic intracellular accumulation fluid in lens fibers and can result in rapid formation of cortical lens opacities in the setting of uncontrolled hyperglycemia, as is often observed in young diabetic patients (Varma, 1980). Additionally, increased glucose levels in the aqueous are thought to cause glycation of lens proteins, leading to increased levels of free radicals (Hong et al, 2000; Stitt, 2005). The glycation is then worsened by the impaired ability of the diabetic lens to handle oxidative stress (Hong et al, 2000; Olofsson et al, 2009). This increased oxidative stress may lead to the subsequent formation of nuclear and mixed-type cataracts (Varma et al, 2010; Richter, 2012).

4.9. Corticosteroids

Corticosteroid use is associated with posterior subcapsular cataracts (Hodge et al, 1995).

4.10. Genetics

Lens-specific genes include gene encoding proteins for growth and transformation of lens fiber cells (cystallins) and mediation of cellular respiration and metabolism, such as major intrinsic polypeptide (MIP) and certain connexins (Agre et al, 1993; Dahm et al, 1999). Mutations in lens-specific genes are associated with hereditary cataracts, possibly through a mechanism which produces a protein interfering with normal proteins, thus disrupting normal function and cataract formation (Beebe et al, 2003).

Numerous hereditary syndromes manifest cataracts as a characteristic feature. Gene mutations are identified for some syndromes: Lowe's syndrome, neurofibromatosis type 2, galactosemia, and Werner syndrome (Litt et al, 1998; Mackay et al, 1999). In most diseases, identifying the genes responsible for the development of the cataract offers no explanation as to why cataracts manifest (Beebe et al, 2003). A better understanding of biochemical and molecular mechanisms underlying cataract formation may provide more information (Kannabiran et al, 2000; Francis et al, 2004).

Recent developments in cataract epidemiology have identified a strong genetic component. Population-based studies have implicated dominant genes in the development of cortical cataracts; genetics also plays a role in nuclear cataracts (Hammond et al, 2000). Increased or decreased gene expression of a few groups of genes in the lens epithelial cells may play an important role in cataract formation. Of the genes whose expression is increased in cataract, many are associated with ionic transport and extracellular matrix proteins, e.g., calcium-ATPase controls calcium channels, copine III is involved in calcium binding, and adducin, a cytoskeletal protein, interacts with epithelial sodium channels. Extracellular matrix proteins include claudin, a component of tight junction filaments that binds adjacent epithelial cells; supervillin, bamacan, and osteonectin are also increased (Hawse et al, 2004; Yanoff and Duker, 2009).

But most genes involved in cataract formation show decreased expression. These genes function in diverse processes including protein synthesis, oxidative stress, structural proteins, chaperones, and cell cycle control proteins. Many of these processes represent metabolic systems designed to preserve lens homeostasis and their decreased expression may reflect the inability of the lens to maintain its internal environment in the presence of stress and/or cataract. Specific examples of these genes include those for: multiple ribosomal protein subunits involved in protein synthesis, which are decreased in cataract relative to clear human lenses; selenoprotein W1, a glutathione-dependent antioxidant which could play a role in defending the lens against oxidative stress; glutathione peroxidases and important oxidative stress enzymes, which are likely to play major roles in lens protection and maintenance; multiple crystallins and other lens structural components; heat shock proteins; and α-crystallin, which in addition to its structural role in the lens, is also a small heat shock protein that can prevent protein aggregation in the lens. Individual changes in gene expression are informative, but further gene identification is needed to define those functional gene clusters that could elucidate major pathways associated with cataract (Hawse et al, 2004; Yanoff and Duker, 2009).

Despite increasing evidence of a genetic component to the development of cataracts, no genes have been identified that are associated with any form of isolated, adult onset cataract. It is likely that multiple loci will be involved. Genetic studies might identify people at greater risk for cataract, who could then modify behaviors (smoking, sun exposure) known to contribute to lens opacity. At present nothing can be done to alter an individual's genetic make-up in relation to cataract. In the future, identification of the genes controlling age-related cataract may facilitate the repair of specific abnormalities at critical loci or may result in the discovery of specific anticataract agents (Congdon, 2001).

4.11. Health

A high body mass index in humans increases the risk of developing posterior subcapsular, nuclear, and cortical cataracts (Hiller et al, 1998). Severe diarrhea and dehydration have also been associated with an increased risk of developing cataracts in some studies (Minassian et al, 1989), but not in others (Mohan et al, 1989), and severe protein-calorie malnutrition is more common in people with cataract (Chaterjee et al, 19820.

4.12. Myopia

The relationship between refractive errors and cataracts has been difficult to establish because of inconsistencies in definitions, populations studied, and methods. After controlling for age, gender, and other cataract risk factors (diabetes, smoking, and education), posterior subcapsular cataracts were found to be associated with myopia, deeper anterior chambers, and longer vitreous chambers, suggesting that the refractive association with posterior subcapsular cataract is axial.

Myopia has been suggested in several cross-sectional epidemiology studies to be associated with the presence of nuclear lens opacities (Leske et al, 2002; Richter et al, 2012). The absence of this relationship in one recent longitudinal study (Richter et al, 2012), as well as the lack of association with axial length, suggests that the previously described relationship may be entirely related to the myopia induced by nuclear sclerosis rather than any causal effect of preexisting myopia on the development of nuclear sclerosis (Wong et al, 2003; Richter et al, 2012).

4.13. Trauma

Blunt trauma, which does not result in rupture of the capsule, may cause an anterior and/or posterior subcapsular cataract, or both. Initially, fluid influx causes swelling and thickening of the lens fibers. Later the fibers become less swollen; the anterior subcapsular region whitens and may develop a characteristic flower-shaped pattern, or an amorphous or punctate opacity. A Vossius ring of iris pigment may be present on the anterior capsule. If the capsule is ruptured, it usually ruptures posteriorly; the lens is rapidly hydrated forming a white cataract. A small capsular penetrating injury may result in localized lens opacity. A larger rupture results in rapid hydration and complete opacification. Penetrating injuries can be caused by accidental or surgical trauma such as a peripheral iridectomy or during a vitrectomy.

Electric shocks as a result of lightning or an industrial accident cause coagulation of proteins or osmotic changes. These cataracts are typically fern-like with grayish white anterior and posterior subcapsular opacities (Fraunfelder and Hanna, 1972). A source of ionizing radiation, such as from x-rays, damages the capsular epithelial cell DNA, affecting protein and enzyme transcription and cell mitosis. An enlarging posterior pole plaque develops. Nonionizing radiation, such as infrared, is the cause of cataract in glassblowers and furnace workers working without protective lenses. A localized rise in the temperature of the iris pigment epithelium causes a characteristic posterior subcapsular cataract, which may be associated with exfoliation of the anterior capsule. The effect of ultraviolet light has been discussed above.

4.14. Other Factors that Increase the Risk of Cataracts Include

- Systemic disorders (Galactosemia, Fabry's disease, Lowe's or oculocerebrorenal syndrome, Alport's syndrome, dystrophia myotonia, Rothmund-Thompson syndrome, Werner's syndrome, Cockayne's syndrome);
- Dermatological disorders (atopic dermatitis and eczema, ichthyosis, incontyinentyia pigmenti);
- Central nervous system disorders (Neurofibromatosis type II, Zellweger syndrome, Norrie's disease);
- Ocular diseases (inflammatory uveitis such as Fuchs' heterochromic cyclitis and juvenile idiopathic arthritis; infective uveitis such as ocular herpes zoster, toxoplasmosis, syphilis, sarcoidosis and tuberculosis; retinitis pigmentosa, Usher's syndrome, gyrate atrophy; anterior segment ischemia).

References

Age-Related Eye Disease Study Research Group. A randomized, placebo-controlled, clinical trial of high-dose supplementation with vitamins C and E and beta carotene for age-related cataract and vision loss: AREDS report no. 9. *Arch Ophthalmol*, 2001; 119, 1439–1452.

Age-Related Eye Disease Study Research Group. Risk factors associated with age-related nuclear and cortical cataract: a case-control study in the Age-Related Eye Disease Study. AREDS report no. 5. *Ophthalmology*, 2001; 108, 1400–1408.

Age-Related Eye Disease Study Research Group. The age-related eye disease study (AREDS) system for classifying cataracts from photographs: AREDS report no. 4. *Am J Ophthalmol*, 2001; 131, 167–175.

Agre, P; Sasaki, S; et al. Aquaporins: a family of water channel proteins. *Am J Physiol*, 1993; 265(3 Pt 2), F461.

Amaya, L; Taylor, D; Russell-Eggitt, I; Nischal, KK; Lengyel, D. The morphology and natural history of childhood cataracts. *Surv Ophthalmol*, 2003; 48, 125-144.

American Academy of Ophthalmology (AAO), Basic and Clinical Science Course. Section 11: Lens and Cataract, 2010-2011.

Ates, O; Alp, HH; Kocer, I; et al. Oxidative DNA damage in patients with cataract. *Acta Ophthalmol*, 2010; 88, 891–895.

Banerjee, KK; Marimuthu, P; Sarkar, A; Chaudhuri, RN. Influence of cigarette smoking on vitamin C, glutathione and lipid peroxidation status. *Indian J Public Health*, 1998; 42, 20 –23.

Beebe, D. The lens. In: Kaufman PL, Adler FH Eds. Adler's Physiology of the Eye: Clinical Application, Tenth Edition. St. Louis: Mosby; 2003, 117-58.

Beebe, DC; Holekamp, NM; Shui, YB. Oxidative damage and the prevention of age-related cataracts. *Ophthalmic Res*, 2010; 44, 155–1 65.

Bollinger, KE; Langston, RH. What can patients expect from cataract surgery? *Cleveland Clinic journal of medicine*, 2008; 75, 193–196.

Boscia, F; Grattagliano, I; Vendemiale, G, et al. Protein oxidation and lens opacity in humans. *Invest Ophthalmol Vis Sci*, 2000; 41, 2461–2465.

Bradbury, BD; Lash, TL; Kaye, JA; Jick, SS. Tamoxifen and cataracts: a null association. *Breast Cancer Res Treat*, 2004; 87, 189–196.

Buch, H; Vinding, T; La Cour, M; Nielsen, NV. The prevalence and causes of bilateral and unilateral blindness in an elderly urban Danish population. The Copenhagen City Eye Study. *Acta Ophthalmol Scand*, 2001; 79, 441-449.

Burke, JP; O'Keefe, M; Bowell, R; Naughten, ER. Ophthalmic findings in classical galactosemia: a screened population. *J Pediatr Ophthalmol Strabismus*, 1989; 26, 165–168.

Cekic, O. Effect of cigarette smoking on copper, lead, and cadmium accumulation in human lens. *Br J Ophthalmol*, 1998; 82, 186–188.

Chang, JR; Koo, E; Agron, E; et al, Age-Related Eye Disease Study Group. Risk factors associated with incident cataracts and cataract surgery in the Age-Related Eye Disease Study (AREDS): AREDS report number 32. *Ophthalmology*, 2011; 118, 2113–2119.

Chaterjee, A; Milton, RC; Thyle, S. Cataract prevalence and aetiology in Punjab. *Br J Ophthalmology*, 1982; 66, 35-42.

Christen, WG; Manson, JE; Seddon, JM; et al. A prospective study of cigarette smoking and risk of cataract in men. *JAMA*, 1992; 268, 989–993.

Chylack, LT, Jr; Wolfe, JK; Singer, DM; et al. The Lens Opacities Classification System III. The Longitudinal Study of Cataract Study Group. *Arch Ophthalmol*, 1993; 111, 831-836.

Congdon, N; O'Colmain, B; Klaver, CC; et al. Causes and prevalence of visual impairment among adults in the United States. *Arch Ophthalmol*, 2004; 122, 477-485.

Congdon, N; Vingerling, JR; Klein, BE; et al. Prevalence of cataract and pseudophakia/aphakia among adults in the United States. *Arch Ophthalmol*, 2004; 122, 487-494.

Congdon, NG. Prevention strategies for age related cataract: present limitations and future possibilities. *Br J Ophthalmol*, 2001; 5, 516-520.

Cruickshanks, KF; Klein, BE; Klein, R. Ultraviolet light exposure and lens opacities: the Beaver Dam Eye Study. *Am J Public Health*, 1992; 82, 1658–1662.

Cumming, RG; Mitchell, P. Hormone replacement therapy, reproductive factors, and cataract. The Blue Mountains Eye Study. *Am J Epidemiol*, 1997; 145, 242-249.

Dahm, R; van Marle, J; et al. Gap junctions containing alpha8-connexin (MP70) in the adult mammalian lens epithelium suggests a re-evaluation of its role in the lens. *Exp Eye Res*, 1999; 69, 45-56.

Delcourt, C; Cristol, JP; Tessier, F; et al, POLA Study Group. Risk factors for cortical, nuclear, and posterior sub-capsular cataracts: the POLA study. *Am J Epidemiol*, 2000; 151, 497–504.

Dobson, R. Ozone depletion will bring big rise in number of cataracts. *BMJ*, 2005; 331 (7528), 1292–1295.

Flynn, HW Jr; Smiddy, WE; eds. Diabetes and Ocular Disease: Past, Present, and Future Therapies. Ophthalmology Monograph 14. San Francisco: *American Academy of Ophthalmology*, 2000, 49-53, 226.

Francis, PJ; Moore, AT. Genetics of childhood cataract. *Curr Opin Ophthalmol*, 2004; 15, 10-15.

Fraunfelder, FT; Fraunfelder, FW. *Drug-Induced Ocular Side Effects*. 5th ed. Boston: Butterworth-Heinemann; 2001.

Fraunfelder, FT; Hanna, C. Electric cataracts. 1: Sequential changes, unusual and prognostic findings. *Arch Ophthalmol*, 1972; 87, 179-183.

Gibson, JM; Rosenthal, AR; Lavery, J. A study of the prevalence of eye disease in the elderly in an English community. *Trans Ophthalmol Soc U K*, 1985, 104, 196-203.

Gill, D; Klose, R; Munier, FL; McFadden, M; Priston, M; Billingsley, G; Ducrey, N; Schorderet, DF; Héon, E. Genetic heterogeneity of the Coppock-like cataract: a mutation in CRYBB2 on chromosome 22q11.2. *Invest Ophthalmol Vis Sci*, 2000; 41, 159-165.

Gillies, MC; Kuzniarz, M; Craig, J; Ball, M; Luo, W; Simpson, JM. Intravitreal triamcinolone-induced elevated intraocular pressure is associated with the development of posterior subcapsular cataract. *Ophthalmology*, 2005; 112, 139–143.

Gold, DH; Weingeist, TA; eds. *The Eye in Systemic Disease*. Philadelphia: Lippincott; 1990, 90, 330–331, 390, 434.

Greiner, J; Chylack, L. Posterior subcapsular cataracts: histopathologic study of steroid-associated cataracts. *Arch Ophthalmol*, 1979; 97, 135–144.

Hammond, CJ; Snieder, H; Spector, TD; Gilbert, CE. Genetic and environmental factors in age-related nuclear cataracts in monozygotic and dizygotic twins. *N Engl J Med*, 2000; 342, 1786–1790.

Hawse, JR; Hejtmancik, JF; Horwitz, J; Kantorow, M. Identification and functional clustering of global gene expression differences between age-related cataract and clear human lenses and aged human lenses. *Exp Eye Res*, 2004; 79, 935-940.

Heck, DE; Gerecke, DR; et al. Solar ultraviolet radiation as a trigger of cell signal transduction. *Toxicol Appl Pharmacol*, 2004; 195, 288-297.

Hejtmancik, JF; Kantorow, M. Molecular genetics of age-related cataract. *Exp Eye Res*, 2004; 79, 3-9.

Hennis, A; Wu, SY; Nemesure, B; Leske, MC. Barbados Eye Studies Group. Risk factors for incident cortical and posterior subcapsular lens opacities in the Barbados Eye Studies. *Arch Ophthalmol*, 2004; 122, 525–530.

Héon, E; Priston, M; Schorderet, DF; Billingsley, GD; Girard, PO; Lubsen, N; Munier, FL. The gamma-crystallins and human cataracts: a puzzle made clearer. *Am J Hum Genet*, 1999; 65, 1261-1267.

Heys, KR; Friedrich, MG; Truscott, RJ. Presbyopia and heat: changes associated with aging of the human lens suggest a functional role for the small heat shock protein, alpha-crystallin, in maintaining lens flexibility. *Aging Cell*, 2007; 6, 807–815.

Hiller, R; Podgor, MJ; Sperduto, RD; et al. A longitudinal study of body mass index and lens opacities. The Framingham Studies. *Ophthalmology*, 1998; 105, 1244–1250.

Hiller, R; Sperduto, RD; Podgor, MJ; et al. Cigarette smoking and the risk of development of lens opacities: the Framingham studies. *Arch Ophthalmol*, 1997; 115, 1113–1118.

Hiratsuka, Y; Li, G. Alcohol and eye diseases: a review of epidemiologic studies. *J Stud Alcohol*, 2001; 62, 397-402.

Hodge, WG; Whitcher, JP; et al. Risk factors for age-related cataracts. *Epidemiol Rev*, 1995; 17, 336-346.

Holmes, JM; Leske, DA; Burke, JP; Hodge, DO. Birth prevalence of visually significant infantile cataract in a defined U.S. population. *Ophthalmic Epidemiol*, 2003; 10, 67-74.

Hong, SB; Lee, KW; Handa, JT; Joo, CK. Effect of advanced glycation end products on lens epithelial cells in vitro. *Biochem Biophys Res Commun*, 2000; 275, 53–59.

Howard, DJ; Ota, RB; Briggs, LA; et al. Environmental tobaccosmoke in the workplace induces oxidative stress in employees, including increased production of 8-hydroxy-2'-deoxyguanosine. *Cancer Epidemiol Biomarkers Prev*, 1998; 7, 141–146.

Irvine, JA; Smith, RE. Lens injuries. In: Shingleton BJ, Hersh PS, Kenyon KR, eds. *Eye Trauma*. St Louis: Mosby; 1991, 126–135.

Iwase, A; Arale, M, Tomidookoro A, et al. Prevalence and causes of low vision and blindness in a Japanese adult population: the Tajimi Study. *Ophthalmology*, 2006; 113, 1354-1362.

Jaffe, GJ; Martin, D; Callanan, D; et al. Fluocinolone acetonide implant (Retisert) for noninfectious posterior uveitis: thirty-four-week results of a multicenter randomized clinical study. *Ophthalmology*, 2006; 113, 1020–1027.

Jobling, AI; Augusteyn, RC. What causes steroid cataracts? A review of steroid-induced posterior subcapsular cataracts. *Clin Exp Optom*, 2002; 85, 61-75.

Kannabiran, C; Balasubramanian, D. Molecular genetics of cataract. *Indian J Ophthalmol*, 2000; 48, 5-13.
Kanski, JJ. Clinical ophthalmology. Fourth edition. *Edinburgh, Butterworth-Heinhemann*, 2002, 673.
Kelly, SP; Thornton, J; Edwards, R; et al. Smoking and cataract: Review of causal association. *J Cataract Refract Surg*, 2005; 31, 2395-2404.
Kiernan, DF; Mieler, WF. The use of intraocular corticosteroids. *Expert Opin Pharmacother*, 2009; 10, 2511–2525.
Klein, BE; Klein, R; et al. Incidence of age-related cataract over a 10-year interval: the Beaver Dam Eye Study. *Ophthalmology*, 2002; 109, 2052-2057.
Klein, BE; Klein, R; et al. Socioeconomic and lifestyle factors and the 10-year incidence of age-related cataracts. *Am J Ophthalmol*, 2003; 136, 506-512.
Klein, BE; Klein, R; Lee, KE; Grady, LM. Statin use and incident nuclear cataract. *JAMA*, 2006; 295, 2752–2758.
Klein, BE; Klein, R; Linton, KL; et al. Assessment of cataracts from photographs in the Beaver Dam Eye Study. *Ophthalmology*, 1990; 97, 1428-1433.
Klein, BE; Klein, R; Moss, SE. Incident cataract surgery: the Beaver Dam eye study. *Ophthalmology*, 1997; 104, 573-580.
Klein, BE; Klein, R; Wang, Q; Moss, SE. Older-onset diabetes and lens opacities: the Beaver Dam Eye Study. *Ophthalmic Epidemiol*, 1995; 2, 49–55.
Klein, BE; Klein, R. Cataracts and macular degeneration in older Americans. *Arch Ophthalmol,* 1982, 100, 571-573.
Klein, BK; Klein, R; Lee, KE; Meuer, SM. Socioeconomic and lifestyle factors and the 10-year incidence of age-related cataracts. *Am J Ophthalmol*, 2003; 136, 506 –512.
Leibowitz, HM; Krueger, DE; Maunder, LR; Milton, RC; Kini, MM; Kahn, HA; Nickerson, RJ; Pool, J; Colton, TL; Ganley, JP; et al. The Framingham Eye Study monograph: An ophthalmological and epidemiological study of cataract, glaucoma, diabetic retinopathy, macular degeneration, and visual acuity in a general population of 2631 adults, 1973–1975. *Surv Ophthalmol,* 1980, 24(Suppl), 335-610.
Leske, MC; Chylack, LT Jr; He, Q; et al. LSC Group. Risk factors for nuclear opalescence in a longitudinal study. *Am J Epidemiol*, 1998; 147, 36–41.
Leske, MC; Wu, SY; Hennis, A; et al, Barbados Eye Study Group. Diabetes, hypertension, and central obesity as cataract risk factors in a black population: the Barbados Eye Study. *Ophthalmology*, 1999; 106, 35– 41.

Leske, MC; Wu, SY; Nemesure, B; Hennis, A. Barbados Eye Studies Group. Risk factors for incident nuclear opacities. *Ophthalmology*, 2002; 109, 1303-1308.

Lewis, A; Congdon, N; Munoz, B; et al. Cataract surgery and subtype in a defined, older population: the SEECAT Project. *Br J Ophthalmol*, 2004; 88, 1512-1517.

Liang, YB; Friedman, DS; Wong, TY; Zhan, SY; Sun, LP; et al. Prevalence and causes of low vision and blindness in a rural Chinese adult population: the Handan Eye study. *Ophthalmology*, 2008; 115, 1965-1972.

Liebman, JM; Ritch, R. Glaucoma secondary to lens intumescence and dislocation. In: Ritch R, Shields MB, Krupin T, eds. *The Glaucomas* 2nd ed. St Louis: Mosby; 1996.

Limburg, H; Barria von-Bischhoffshausen, F; Gomez, P; Silva, JC; Foster, A. Review of recent surveys on blindness and visual impairment in Latin America. *Br J Ophthalmol*, 2008; 92, 316-319.

Lipman, RM; Tripathi, BJ; Tripathi, RC. Cataracts induced by microwave and ionizing radiation. *Surv Ophthalmol*, 1988; 33, 200–210.

Litt, M; Kramer, P; et al. Autosomal dominant congenital cataract associated with a missense mutation in the human alpha crystallin gene CRYAA. *Hum Mol Genet*, 1998; 7, 471-474.

Mackay, D; Ionides, A; et al. Connexin46 mutations in autosomal dominant congenital cataract. *Am J Hum Genet*, 1999; 64, 1357-1364.

Magno, BV; Freidlin, V; Datiles, MB. 3rd. Reproducibility of the NEI Scheimpflug Cataract Imaging System. *Invest Ophthalmol Vis Sci*, 1994; 35, 3078-3084.

Mannis, MJ; Macsai, MS; Huntley, AC; eds. *Eye and Skin Disease*. Philadelphia: Lippincott-Raven; 1996.

Marbeley, DA; Hollands; Chuo, J; Tam, G; et al. The prevalence of low vision and blindness in Canada. *Eye* (Lond), 2006; 20, 341-346.

McCarty, CA; Taylor, HR. A review of the epidemiologic evidence linking ultraviolet radiation and cataracts. *Dev Ophthalmol*, 2002; 35, 21-31.

McCarty, CA; Taylor, HR. The genetics of cataract. *Invest Ophthalmol Vis Sci*, 2001; 42, 1677-1678.

McCarty, CA; Nanjan, MB; Taylor, HR. Attributable risk estimates for cataract to prioritize medical and public health action. *Invest Ophthalmol Vis Sci*, 1999; 41, 3720-3725.

Minassian, DC; Mehra, V; Verry, JD. Dehydrational crisis: a major risk factor in blinding cataract. *Br J Ophthalmol*, 1989; 73, 100-105.

Morris, MS; Jacques, PF; Hankinson, SE; et al. Moderate alcoholic beverage intake and early nuclear and cortical lens opacities. *Ophthalmic Epidemiol*, 2004; 11, 53-65.

Neale, RE; Purdie, JL; Hirst, LW; Green, AC. Sun exposure as a risk factor for nuclear cataract. *Epidemiology*, 2003; 14, 707-712.

Nicholl, ID; Stitt, AW; Moore, JE; et al. Increased levels of advanced glycation endproducts in the lenses and blood vessels of cigarette smokers. *Mol Med*, 1998; 4, 594–601.

Nirmalan, PK; Robin, AL; et al. Risk factors for age related cataract in a rural population of southern India: the Aravind Comprehensive Eye Study. *Br J Ophthalmol*, 2004; 88, 989-994.

Ottonello, S; Foroni, C; Carta, A; Petrucco, S; Maraini, G. Oxidative stress and age-related cataract. *Ophthalmologica*, 2000; 214, 78-85.

Palmquist, BM; Philipson, B; Barr, PO. Nuclear cataract and myopia during hyperbaric oxygen therapy. *Br J Ophthalmol*, 1984; 68, 113–117.

Panchapakesan, J; Mitchell, P; Tumuluri, K; et al. Five year incidence of cataract surgery: the Blue Mountains Eye Study. *Br J Ophthalmol*, 2003; 87, 168-172.

Pokhrel, AK; Smith, KR; Khalakdina, A, et al. Case-control study of indoor cooking smoke exposure and cataract in Nepal and India. *Int J Epidemiol*, 2005; 34, 702–708.

Portellos, M; Orlin, SE; Kozart, DM. Electric cataracts [photo essay]. *Arch Ophthalmol*, 1996; 114, 1022–1023.

Rafnsson, V; Olafsdottir, E; Hrafnkelsson, J; Sasaki, H; Arnarsson, A; Jonasson, F. Cosmic radiation increases the risk of nuclear cataract in airline pilots: a population-based case-control study. *Arch Ophthalmol*, 2005; 123, 1102–1105.

Ramakrishnan, S; Sulochana, KN; Selvaraj, T; et al. Smoking of beedies and cataract: cadmium and vitamin C in the lens and blood. *Br J Ophthalmol*, 1995; 79, 202–20 6.

Reddy, MA; Francis, PJ; Berry, V; Bhattacharya, SS; Moore, AT. Molecular genetic basis of inherited cataract and associated Figure 3. Forward and reverse sequence analyses of the affected and phenotypes. *Surv Ophthalmol*, 2004; 49, 300-315.

Resnikoff, S; Pascolini, D; Etya'ale, D; et al. Global data on visual impairment in the year 2002. *Bull World Health Org*, 2004; 82, 844-851.

Richter, C; Epstein, DL. Lens-induced open-angle glaucoma. In: Ritch R, Shields MB, Krupin T, eds. *The Glaucomas*. 2nd ed. St Louis: Mosby; 1996.

Richter, GM; Choudhury, F; Mina Torres, M; Azen, SP; Rohit Varma, R; for the Los Angeles Latino Eye Study Group. Risk Factors for Incident Cortical, Nuclear, Posterior Subcapsular, and Mixed Lens Opacities. The Los Angeles Latino Eye Study. *Ophthalmology,* 2012; 119, 2040–2047.

Richter, GM; Torres, M; Choudhury, F; et al, Los Angeles Latino Eye Study Group. Risk factors for cortical, nuclear, posterior subcapsular, and mixed lens opacities: the Los Angeles Latino Eye Study. *Ophthalmology,* 2012; 119, 547–554.

Sarma, U; Brunner, E; et al. Nutrition and the epidemiology of cataract and age-related maculopathy. *Eur J Clin Nutr,* 1994; 48, 1-8.

Schlienger, RG; Haefeli, WE; Jick, H; Meier, CR. Risk of cataract in patients treated with statins. *Arch Intern Med,* 2001; 161, 2021–2026.

Schlötzer-Schrehardt, U; Naumann, GO. Ocular and systemic pseudoexfoliation syndrome. *Am J Ophthalmol,* 2006; 141, 921–937.

Shiels, A; Hejtmancik, JF. Genetic origins of cataract. *Arch Ophthalmol,* 2007; 25, 165-173.

Sliney, DH. UV radiation ocular exposure dosimetry. *Doc Ophthalmol,* 1994; 88 (3-4), 243–254.

Spencer, R; Andelman, S. Steroid cataracts. Posterior subcapsular cataract formation in rheumatoid arthritis patients on long term steroid therapy. *Arch Ophthalmol,* 1965; 74, 38–41.

Stitt, AW. The Maillard reaction in eye diseases. *Ann N Y Acad Sci,* 2005; 1043, 582–597.

Takahashi, A; Masuda, A; Sun, M; et al. Oxidative stressinduced apoptosis is associated with alterations in mitochondrial caspase activity and Bcl-2-dependent alterations in mitochondrial pH (pHm). *Brain Res Bull,* 2004; 62, 497–504.

Tan, JS; Wang, JJ; Younan, C; et al. Smoking and the long-term incidence of cataract: the Blue Mountains Eye Study. *Ophthalmic Epidemiol,* 2008; 15, 155– 161.

Taylor, HR; West, SK. The clinical grading of lens opacities. *Aust N Z J Ophthalmol,* 1989; 17, 81-86.

Taylor, A. *Nutritional and environmental influences on risk for cataract.* In: Tasman W., Jaeger E.A., ed. *Duane's clinical ophthalmology,* vol 1, Ch, Philadelphia: Lippincott Williams and Wilkins; 2002.

Truscott, RJ. Age-related nuclear cataract– oxidation is the key. *Exp Eye Res,* 2005; 80, 709 –725.

Urban, RC Jr; Cotlier, E. Corticosteroid-induced cataracts. *Surv Ophthalmol,* 1986; 31, 102–110.

van den Brûle, J; Degueldre, F; Galand, A. "[Drug-induced cataracts]" (in French). *Revue médicale de Liège*, 1998; 53, 766–769.

Vanita Singh, JR; Singh, D. Genetic and segregation analysis of congenital cataract in the Indian population. *Clin Genet*, 1999; 56, 389-393.

Varma, R; Richter, GM; Torres, M; et al. Los Angeles Latino Eye Study Group. Four-year incidence and progression of lens opacities: the Los Angeles Latino Eye Study. *Am J Ophthalmol*, 2010; 149, 728 –734.

Varma, R; Torres, M. Prevalence of lens opacities in Latinos: the Los Angeles Latino Eye Study. *Ophthalmology*, 2004; 111, 1449-1456.

Varma, SD. Aldose reductase and the etiology of diabetic cataracts. *Curr Top Eye Res*, 1980; 3, 91–155.

Ventura, L; Lam, KW; Lin, TY. The differences between brunescent and opalescent nucleosclerosis. *Lens Research*, 1987; 4, 79-86.

Vinson, JA. Oxidative stress in cataracts. *Pathophysiology*, 2006; 13, 151-162.

Vivino, MA; Chintalagiri, S; Trus, B; Datiles, M. Development of a Scheimpflug slit lamp camera system for quantitative densitometric analysis. *Eye*, 1993; 7 (Pt 6), 791-798.

Waagbo, R; Hamre, K; et al. Cataract formation in Atlantic salmon, Salmo salar L, smolt relative to dietary pro- and antioxidants and lipid level. *J Fish Dis*, 2003; 26, 213-229.

Wang, S; Wang, JJ; Wong, TY. Alcohol and eye diseases. *Surv Ophthalmol*, 2008: 53, 512–525.

West, S; Munoz, B; Emmett, EA; Taylor, HR. Cigarette smoking and risk of nuclear cataracts. *Arch Ophthalmol*, 1989; 107, 1166–1169.

West, SK; Duncan, DD; Muñoz, B; et al. Sunlight exposure and risk of lens opacities in a population-based study: the Salisbury Eye Evaluation Project. *JAMA*, 1998; 280, 714–718.

West, SK; Valmadrid, CT. Epidemiology of risk factors for age-related cataract. *Surv Ophthalmol*, 1995; 39, 323–334.

Winkler, BS; Orselli, SM; et al. The redox couple between glutathione and ascorbic acid: a chemical and physiological perspective. *Free Radic Biol Med*, 1994; 17, 333-349.

Wong, TY; Foster, PJ; Johnson, GJ; et al. Refractive errors, axial ocular dimensions, and age-related cataracts: The Tanjong Pagar Survey. *Invest Ophthalmol Vis Sci*, 2003; 44, 1479-1485.

Worgul, BV; Merriam, GR; et al. Lens epithelium and radiation cataract. I. Preliminary studies. *Arch Ophthalmol*, 1976; 94, 996-999.

Yanoff, M; Duker, JS. Ophthalmology. Third edition. *Philadelpia, Mosby Elsevier*, 2009. 1528.

You, QS; XU, L; Yang, YX; Jonas, JB. Five-year incidence of visual impairment and blindness in adult Chinese: the Beijing Eye Study. *Ophthalmology*, 2011; 118, 1069-1075.

Zenkel, M; Lewczuk, P; Jünemann, A; Kruse, FE; Naumann, GO; Schlötzer-Schrehardt, U. Proinflammatory cytokines are involved in the initiation of the abnormal matrix process in pseudoexfoliation syndrome/glaucoma. *Am J Pathol*, 2010; 176, 2868–2879. Epub 2010 A.

Zhang, Y; Zhang, L; Sun, D; et al. Genetic polymorphisms of superoxide dismutases, catalase, and glutathione peroxidase in age-related cataract. *Mol Vis* [serial online] 2011; 17, 2325–2332. Available at: http://www.molvis.org/molvis/v17/a253/. Accessed April 19, 2012.

In: Cataracts and Cataract Surgery
Editor: Didier Navarro

ISBN: 978-1-62808-400-9
© 2013 Nova Science Publishers, Inc.

Chapter III

A Practical Guide to the Management of Intraoperative Floppy Iris Syndrome (IFIS)

Allan Storr-Paulsen[*]
Consultant Senior Ophthalmic Surgeon, Koge Eye Clinic,
Koge, Denmark

Abstract

Intraocular floppy iris syndrome (IFIS) observed during cataract surgery includes fluttering and billowing of the iris, a propensity for iris prolapse though incisions, and constriction of the pupil leading to higher rates of complications. Although IFIS may have a multifactorial background, it is most often associated with the chronic use of systemic sympathetic α-1 AR antagonists, and tamsulosin in particular. But many other drugs, and even alternative medicine have been reported to cause a floppy iris. Management of IFIS includes preoperative precautions such as thorough questioning of the medical history, and α-1a antagonists in particular. Moreover, we propose a surgical strategy including the use of a high viscous viscoelastic, the use of pupil expansions rings, and to keep phenylephrine ready for intracameral injection in case of a progressive pupil constriction during surgery.

---

[*] Email: allan.storr@gmail.com.

Introduction

Intraoperative floppy iris syndrome (IFIS) seen in cataract surgery was described in 2005 (Chang & Campbell 2005; Parssinen 2005). IFIS is characterized by billowing of the iris stroma in response to normal irrigation currents, a propensity for the floppy iris to prolapse through the incisions, and a progressive pupillary constriction during the phaco procedure. The extent of the clinical presentation varies widely, from a mild form with only a fluttering iris, to a more severe form with the complete triad (Chang et al. 2007).

In cataract surgery, a well dilated pupil and stable iris plate is crucial to a safe and uncomplicated operation. An adequate pupillary dilatation is achieved with administration of preoperative mydriatic medications, most often topical cyclopentolate 1% combined with phenylephrine 2.5% – 10%. Recent reports recommend a solution with lidocaine, cyclopentolate, and phenylephrine injected intracamerally at the beginning of the operation without preoperative mydriatica (Lundberg & Behndig 2003).

In this chapter, general management and guidelines of IFIS will be presented.

Epidemiology

The prevalence of IFIS in cataract patients varies from 0.5%-1.6% in the UK (Cheung et al. 2006; Chadha et al. 2007), 1.1% in Japan (Oshika et al. 2007), 1.6% in Turkey (Takmaz & Can 2007), and up to 2% in the USA (Chang & Campbell 2005). The incidence of IFIS during cataract surgery in patients on tamsulosin medication varies from 43 – 90% (Cheung et al. 2006; Chadha et al. 2007; Storr-Paulsen et al. 2013). In contrast, the incidence of IFIS in patients taking one of the other α-1a AR (adrenergic receptor) antagonists, e.g. alfuzosin, is only 10-15% (Blouin et al. 2007).

Etiology

Although IFIS may have a multifactorial background, it is most often associated with the chronic use of systemic sympathetic α-1 AR antagonists, and tamsulosin in particular. But many other drugs, and even alternative medicine have been reported to cause a floppy iris (Table 1) (Schwinn &

A Practical Guide to the Management of IFIS 113

Afshari 2006). The main indication for treatment with an α-1 AR antagonist is benign prostatic hyperplasia (BPH) and lower urinary tract symptoms (LUTS) which have a high prevalence in the elderly male population. The prevalence of BPH / LUTS and cataract is similar, and increasing with age.

Table 1. Drugs and diseases with proven or suspect effect on the iris (IFIS)

Medication used in urology:
α-$_1$ AR antagonists (tamsulosin, alfuzosin, doxazosin, terazosin)
5-α-reductase antagonists (fenasteride and dutasteride)

Antipsychotic medicine:
Dopamine D$_2$- receptor antagonists (zuclopenthixol and risperidon)
Antidepressive medicine: α-$_2$ ARs (mianserin)

Anti-Alzheimer medicine:
Acetylcholinesterase antagonists (donepezil, galantamin)

Cardio-vascular diseases:
combined α- and β AR antagonists (labetalol)
Angiotensin-2 and endothelin-1 antagonists
ACE-antagonists: benazepril, captopril, perindopril, tandolapril.

Alternative medicine:
Saw palmetto (Serenoa repens)

The smooth muscles of the human prostate / bladder neck and the iris dilator muscle of the eye are both predominantly stimulated by adrenergic subtype α-1a and (to a lesser extend) α-1d. Therefore, antagonists to α-1a AR relax the muscle tone, which then lead to a decrease in the pressure within the lower urinary tract, improving urinary outflow, and concomitantly, producing relaxation of the iris dilator muscle causing a floppy iris and miosis. Thus, systemic treatment with α-1 AR inhibitors (alfuzosin, doxazosin, tamsulosin and terazosin) has been a successful therapy of LUTS, including BPH, but the treatment may cause some degree of IFIS during cataract surgery. Due to a better cardio-vascular profile, tamsulosin and alfuzosin seem to be tolerated better than doxazosin and terazosin (Djavan et al. 2004). Tamsulosin has a very high affinity for the α-1a and α-1d ARs in the smooth muscular tissue of the iris. Alfuzosin acts clinically in a more uro-selective manner, which might explain, that alfuzosin causes IFIS less frequent than tamsulosin, decreasing the odd ratio for IFIS to 1:32 compared to patients exposed to tamsulosin (Blouin et al. 2007).

IFIS with or without small pupils potentially increases the risk of intraoperative complication, such as iris trauma, zonular dehiscence, posterior capsule rupture, vitreous loss, as well as postoperative complication with increased intraocular pressure and cystoid macular edema (Chang et al. 2007; Nguyen et al. 2007).

Management of IFIS

A) Preoperative Precautions

A thorough questioning of the previous and current medical history is mandatory in all patients undergoing cataract surgery. Of particular interest is an anamnesis of symptoms from the prostate in male, and the lower urinary tract in both gender, as α-1a AR inhibitors may be prescribed for LUTS and arterial hypertension in females as well. IFIS may develop in patients treated with tamsulosin for only a few months. It seems rational to stop the treatment with α-1 AR antagonists preoperatively, but stopping the treatment with tamsulosin can not predict the severity of IFIS, although the preoperative pupil diameter may be larger (Chang et al. 2007; Nguyen et al. 2007).

B) Preoperative Deep Anterior Chamber

In patients with a shallow anterior chamber (AC) there is limited space for phaco manoeuvres, and dilation of the pupil may give an increased IOP. In these cases, we recommend a drinkable glycerol-mixture (glycerol 85%; 59 gram in 100 mL purified water) preoperatively. We use half of the recommended dose of what is recommended a patient with an acute attack of narrow angle glaucoma; i.e. ½ mL per kilo bodyweight. The glycerol is given per os half an hour before surgery. This procedure may increase AC with up to 1-2 mm.

C) Preoperative Dilatation

A preoperative maximum pupillary dilatation is mandatory. We recommend cyclopentolate 1% (an anti-cholinergic / anti-muscarinic drug) to relax the sphincter of the pupil, combined with phenylephrine 2.5% – 10% (an α-1 AR agonist) to enhance the dilatation and increase the tone of the iris dilator stroma administrated twice at 15-20 minutes' interval before surgery. We add a non-steroid anti-inflammatory drug (diclofenac 0.1% / ketorolac 0.5%) to provide a more stable dilatation throughout the surgery. A preoperatively poorly dilated pupil may predict a peroperative increased risk to manifest IFIS. At our affiliation, a preoperative pupil diameter ≤ 6 mm in IFIS patients indicate the need for iris retractors, pupil expansion rings or intracameral phenylephrine.

Atropine 1% applied topically prior to cataract surgery in patients on tamsulosin has been advocated to obtain a maximum preoperative dilatation (Bendel & Phillips 2006; Masket & Belani 2007). In the case series by Bendel & Philips, atropine 1% was prescribed twice daily for 10 days. Thirteen out of 16 patients (81%) on tamsulosin did not require other modification for their cataract surgery. But this treatment regimen represents a risk in an elderly group of patients on α-1 AR medication, due to well-known cardiac and cerebral side-effects.

Masket & Belani used administration of topical atropine 1% three times daily for two days preoperatively in addition to routine preoperative mydriatics. During the operative procedure, 0.3 to 0.5 mL intracameral epinephrine diluted 1:2500 with BSS was placed under the iris. They reported 19 eyes out of 20 to have an excellent pupil dilatation without signs of IFIS.

If the surgeon decides to discontinue the patient's α-1 inhibitor medication prior to surgery, care should be taken with prescription of atropine as preoperative medication due to the risk of intensified urinary problems and even acute urinary retention (Parssinen et al. 2006) (Masket & Belani 2007).

D) Intraoperative Strategies

Several surgical strategies have been proposed for management of the progressive pupillary constriction and the billowing of the iris stroma in IFIS patients:

Epinephrine in the Irrigation Solution

Epinephrine, a combined α- and β AR agonist, should be added to the irrigation solution. We recommend 1 mL epinephrine 1 mg/mL (preservative- and sulfite free) in 1000 mL balanced salt solution (1: 1.000,000) with a pH within the range of 6.5 – 8.5. If intracameral mydriatics are used there is no need for epinephrine irrigation (Lundberg & Behndig 2007).

Incision and Wound Construction

The incision and the wound construction should be created to provide a self-sealing wound with a minimum risk of iris prolapse. Irrigation and aspiration flow rates should be reduced to prevent iris fluttering.

Intracameral Use of Epinephrine

Intracameral injection of unpreserved epinephrine has been suggested by several authors. Myers & Shugar reported good effect of an intracameral mydriatic and anesthetic mixture, the "epi-Shugar" solution, comprised of epinephrine 0.025% and lidocaine 0.75% in BSS Plus. The technique showed excellent results in a paired prospective single masked study (Myers & Shugar 2009). The epi-Shugar solution consists of a 1 : 4,000 epinephrine mixture with a pH of 6.9. There was no report of corneal endothelial cell damage (Shugar 2006). Masket and Belani combined pre-operative topical atropine 1% three times daily for 2 days with intracameral injection of 0.3 – 0.5 mL unpreserved epinephrine diluted 1:2.500 with BSS. They reported a high rate of success in IFIS patients treated with this combined technique (19 out of 20 patients had no signs of IFIS) (Masket & Belani 2007). Takmaz and Can reported the use of a mixture of 0.1 mL unpreserved epinephrine (0.5 mg/mL) diluted with 2 mL BSS (1:4.000). One mL of this solution was then injected into the anterior chamber. They reported no change in the incidence of IFIS, but the mixture seemed effective in order to prevent miosis (Takmaz & Can 2007).

Intracameral Injection of Phenylephrine

Intracameral injection of phenylephrine, an α-1 AR agonist, has been recommended to reverse intraoperative iris fluttering and pupil constriction (Manvikar & Allen 2006; Gurbaxani & Packard 2007). In both studies, diluted phenylephrine 2.5% was used (Minims®, buffered with bisulfite and edetate). Manvikar & Allen used a solution with 0.25 mL unpreserved phenylephrine 2.5% (Minims) diluted with 2 mL BSS. This corresponds to a 1:360 dilution with a pH of 6.4. The authors reported in a study comprising 32 eyes that the solution had a good effect in preventing IFIS. Gurbaxani & Packard reported on the use of intracameral phenylephrine 2.5% mixed with 1 mL BSS in a study with seven patients on tamsulosin. All patients had significant reduction in the signs of IFIS, and a sustained pupillary dilation in all cases. No clinical signs of corneal edema were reported, but the density of endothelial cell was not evaluated.

In an early report by Edelhauser et al., a cytotoxic effect on the endothelium of phenylephrine at a concentration of 2.5% was described in cases where the epithelium was removed (Edelhauser et al. 1979). In a recent report on corneal endothelial cell changes in cataract patients on tamsulosin, we found no association between the intracameral use of 0.25 mL phenylephrine 2.5% (Minims®) in 2 mL BBS and postoperative endothelial cell loss (Storr-Paulsen et al. 2013).

Capsular Staining

Capsular staining with tryptan blue 0.06% (Vision Blue, DORC, The Netherlands) is an excellent way to visualize an obscured leading edge of the capsulorrhexis at the initial stage of the operation due to a small pupil or a mature cataract. Tryptan blue is also very effective to visualize the border of the rhexis, if an iris retractor or a Malyugin ring are required later in the procedure due to progressive miosis. Tryptan blue is safe and effective as an adjunct for capsule visularization (de Waard et al. 2002; Jacobs et al. 2006).

Use of Ophthalmic Viscosurgical Devices (OVDs)

Injection of Healon5 was one of four different surgical strategies used to manage IFIS in a multicenter study. A total of 98 of 103 cases were completed with Healon5 alone and the remaining five cases required additional use of iris retractors / iris expansion rings (Chang et al. 2007). In a survey of surgeons' experiences with IFIS in the UK, 27% of the responding surgeons reported using Healon5, and 85% found it effective (Nguyen et al. 2007).

In 1999, Arshinoff described a technique, where a lower viscosity dispersive OVD was used together with a higher viscosity cohesive OVD (Arshinoff 1999). This "soft-shell" technique is performed with the dispersive injected into the anterior chamber until the chamber is 75-80% full. The cohesive is then injected on the surface of the anterior capsule, pushing the dispersive OVD upward and outward until the pupil stops dilating. The technique was later modified to improve surgery, especially in IFIS patients (Arshinoff 2006).

Use of Iris Retractors

The use of flexible iris retractors to enlarge the pupil was originally described in the early 1990s (de Juan E Jr & Hickingbotham 1991; Nichamin 1993) and later modified to create a diamond shape, which is indeed suitable in IFIS surgery (Oetting & Omphroy 2002). In the UK survey of surgeons' preferences in IFIS cases, 61% of the responders chose iris retractors, and 72% of that group found them effective (Nguyen et al. 2007). In the American multicenter study, iris retractors were only used in 31% of the cases. The difference may be explained by the fact that the British survey questioned all UK eye surgeons about their experiences, whereas the American study only asked 15 selected and highly experienced surgeons (Chang et al. 2007). Pupil stretching and sphincterotomies are usually of no effect because of the elasticity of the pupil margin, and may worsen the constriction of the pupil (Chang & Campbell 2005).

Use of Pupil Expansion Rings

Pupil expansion rings have been used to enlarge the pupil and to maintain the size throughout the surgery. Expansion rings were only used by 3% of the surgeons in the UK survey (Nguyen et al. 2007), and expansion rings were the least used of four alternatives (4% of cases) in the American multicenter study. The disposable Malyugin expansion ring seems to gain increasing popularity in patients taking tamsulosin who present with a preoperative pupil diameter of < 6 mm (Chang 2008).

Conclusion

1) IFIS is strongly associated with chronic use of systemic α-1a AR antagonists, in particular tamsulosin, but other drugs may also contribute to the syndrome. The surgeon should obtain a comprehensive anamnesis of previous and current medications, specially with regard to LUTS and BHP.
2) Preoperative dilation including cyclopentolate, phenylephrine and NSAIDs is important. Atropine 1% may be used, but caution should be taken in elderly patients because of the risk of cardiac side effects and acute urinary retention.
3) A shallow anterior chamber should be deepened by glycerol 85%, 50 – 75 mL given ½ hour before surgery.
4) Epinephrine should be added to the irrigation solution.

5) Capsular staining will facilitate visualization of the rhexis edge.
6) Use a viscoadaptive (Healon5 / Ivisc) during surgery, if necessary in a "soft-shell" fashion.
7) Keep phenylephrine ready for intracameral injection.
8) Consider the use of iris retractors or the Malyugin ring if preoperative dilation is < 6 mm.

References

Arshinoff SA. (1999): Dispersive-cohesive viscoelastic soft shell technique. *J Cataract Refract Surg* 25: 167-173.
Arshinoff SA. (2006): Modified SST-USST for tamsulosin-associated intraoperative [corrected] floppy-iris syndrome. *J Cataract Refract Surg* 32: 559-561.
Bendel RE, Phillips MB. (2006): Preoperative use of atropine to prevent intraoperative floppy-iris syndrome in patients taking tamsulosin. *J Cataract Refract Surg* 32: 1603-1605.
Blouin MC, Blouin J, Perreault S, Lapointe A, Dragomir A. (2007): Intraoperative floppy-iris syndrome associated with alpha1-adrenoreceptors: comparison of tamsulosin and alfuzosin. *J Cataract Refract Surg* 33: 1227-1234.
Chadha V, Borooah S, Tey A, Styles C, Singh J. (2007): Floppy iris behaviour during cataract surgery: associations and variations. *Br J Ophthalmol* 91: 40-42.
Chang DF. (2008): Use of Malyugin pupil expansion device for intraoperative floppy-iris syndrome: results in 30 consecutive cases. *J Cataract Refract Surg* 34: 835-841.
Chang DF, Campbell JR. (2005): Intraoperative floppy iris syndrome associated with tamsulosin. *J Cataract Refract Surg* 31: 664-673.
Chang DF, Osher RH, Wang L, Koch DD. (2007): Prospective multicenter evaluation of cataract surgery in patients taking tamsulosin (Flomax). *Ophthalmology* 114: 957-964.
Cheung CM, Awan MA, Sandramouli S. (2006): Prevalence and clinical findings of tamsulosin-associated intraoperative floppy-iris syndrome. J Cataract Refract *Surg* 32: 1336-1339.
de Juan E Jr, Hickingbotham D. (1991): Flexible iris retractor. *Am J Ophthalmol* 111: 776-777.

de Waard PW, Budo CJ, Melles GR. (2002): Trypan blue capsular staining to "find" the leading edge of a "lost" capsulorhexis. *Am J Ophthalmol* 134: 271-272.

Djavan B, Chapple C, Milani S, Marberger M. (2004): State of the art on the efficacy and tolerability of alpha1-adrenoceptor antagonists in patients with lower urinary tract symptoms suggestive of benign prostatic hyperplasia. *Urology* 64: 1081-1088.

Edelhauser HF, Hine JE, Pederson H, Van Horn DL, Schultz RO. (1979): The effect of phenylephrine on the cornea. *Arch Ophthalmol* 97: 937-947.

Gurbaxani A, Packard R. (2007): Intracameral phenylephrine to prevent floppy iris syndrome during cataract surgery in patients on tamsulosin. *Eye* 21: 331-332.

Jacobs DS, Cox TA, Wagoner MD, Ariyasu RG, Karp CL. (2006): Capsule staining as an adjunct to cataract surgery: a report from the American Academy of Ophthalmology. *Ophthalmology* 113: 707-713.

Lundberg B, Behndig A. (2003): Intracameral mydriatics in phacoemulsification cataract surgery. *J Cataract Refract Surg* 29: 2366-2371.

Lundberg B, Behndig A. (2007): Intracameral mydriatics in phacoemulsification surgery obviate the need for epinephrine irrigation. *Acta Ophthalmol Scand* 85: 546-550.

Manvikar S, Allen D. (2006): Cataract surgery management in patients taking tamsulosin staged approach. *J Cataract Refract Surg* 32: 1611-1614.

Masket S, Belani S. (2007): Combined preoperative topical atropine sulfate 1% and intracameral nonpreserved epinephrine hydrochloride 1:4000 [corrected] for management of intraoperative floppy-iris syndrome. *J Cataract Refract Surg* 33: 580-582.

Myers WG, Shugar JK. (2009): Optimizing the intracameral dilation regimen for cataract surgery: prospective randomized comparison of 2 solutions. *J Cataract Refract Surg* 35: 273-276.

Nguyen DQ, Sebastian RT, Kyle G. (2007): Surgeon's experiences of the intraoperative floppy iris syndrome in the United Kingdom. *Eye* 21: 443-444.

Nichamin LD. (1993): Enlarging the pupil for cataract extraction using flexible nylon iris retractors. *J Cataract Refract Surg* 19: 793-796.

Oetting TA, Omphroy LC. (2002): Modified technique using flexible iris retractors in clear corneal cataract surgery. *J Cataract Refract Surg* 28: 596-598.

Oshika T, Ohashi Y, Inamura M, Ohki K, Okamoto S, Koyama T, Sakabe I, Takahashi K, Fujita Y, et al. (2007): Incidence of intraoperative floppy iris syndrome in patients on either systemic or topical alpha(1)-adrenoceptor antagonist. *Am J Ophthalmol* 143: 150-151.

Parssinen O. (2005): The use of tamsulosin and iris hypotony during cataract surgery. *Acta Ophthalmol Scand* 83: 624-626.

Parssinen O, Leppanen E, Keski-Rahkonen P, Mauriala T, Dugue B, Lehtonen M. (2006): Influence of tamsulosin on the iris and its implications for cataract surgery. *Invest Ophthalmol Vis Sci* 47: 3766-3771.

Schwinn DA, Afshari NA. (2006): alpha(1)-Adrenergic receptor antagonists and the iris: new mechanistic insights into floppy iris syndrome. *Surv Ophthalmol* 51: 501-512.

Shugar JK. (2006): Use of epinephrine for IFIS prophylaxis. *J Cataract Refract Surg* 32: 1074-1075.

Storr-Paulsen A, Skovlund J, Norregaard JC, Thulesen J. (2013): Corneal endothelial cell changes after cataract surgery in patients on systemic sympathetic alpha-1a medication (tamsulosin). *Acta Ophthalmol Scand* 91: In press

Takmaz T, Can I. (2007): Clinical features, complications, and incidence of intraoperative floppy iris syndrome in patients taking tamsulosin. *Eur J Ophthalmol* 17: 909-913.

In: Cataracts and Cataract Surgery
Editor: Didier Navarro

ISBN: 978-1-62808-400-9
© 2013 Nova Science Publishers, Inc.

Chapter IV

A Comparison of Safety and Visual Improvement of Phacoemulsification with Sutureless Single-Port 25-Gauge Vitrectomy versus Phacoemulsication Alone for Eyes with Extremely Shallow Anterior Chambers

Hiroshi Kobayashi[*]
Department of Ophthalmology, Kanmon Medical Center,
Shimonoseki, Japan

Note

There was no commercial sponsorship or support for this study.

---

[*] Corresponding author and address for correspondence: To Hiroshi Kobayashi MD, PhD, Department of Ophthalmology, Kanmon Medical Center, 1-1 Chofu-satoura-cho, Shimonoseki 752-8510, Japan. PHONE: [81] 83-241-1199, FAX: [81] 83-241-1316; E-mail: kobi@earth.ocn.ne.jp.

Abstract

Purpose: To compare the visual improvement and safety of phacoemulsication with suturelss transconjunctival single-port 25-gauge vitrectomy and phacoemulsication for eyes with extremely shallow anterior chamber.

Methods: Forty patients with 2.5 mm or less of the anterior chamber depth who were scheduled to undergo phacoemulsification and intraocular lens implantation were studied. Eyes were assigned randomly to either phacoemulsication with 25-gauge vitrectomy or phacoemulsication alone. Patients were followed-up for 6 months and the incidence of intra- and postoperative complications was compared.

Results: Mean anterior chamber depth was 2.19 ± 0.22 mm in the phacoemulsication with vitrectomy group and 2.17 ± 0.25 mm in the phacoemulsication alone group (P = 0.8). There was no significant difference in the mean best-corrected visual acuity between the groups at any time point before and after surgery. neal endothelial cell density at baseline and at 6 months postoperatively was 2420±360/mm^2 and 2282± 3331/ mm^2 in the phacoemulsication with vitrectomy group and 2436±313/mm^2 and 2248±335/mm^2 in the phacoemulsication alone group, respectively. The phacoemulsication alone group showed a loss of 7.9±3.0 % at 6 months in the change of corneal endothelium cell density, which was significantly greater than that of the phacoemusication with vitrectomy group (P = 0.0057) Complications included two cases (10 %) of continuous curvilinear capsulorhexis tear in the phacoemulsication alone group, whereas two cases (8%) of zonular dehiscence occurred in each group.

Keywords: Phacoemulsification, sutureless single- port vitrectomy, corneal endothelial cell count

Introduction

Although technique of phacoemulsication recently has evolved with the advent of foldable intraocular lens, patients with extremely shallow anterior chamber pose a clinical challenge when therapy needs cataract surgery. Recent studies proposed an application of core vitrectomy before phacoemulsication. [1,2] Theoretically, it may provide reduction of vitreous pressure and allow the anterior chamber deep to facilitate further procedures. Little is known for safety of the vitrectomy prior to phacoemulsification. The aim of this study is to compare the safety and visual improvement of phacoemulsication with sutureless transconjunctival single-port 25-gauge vitrectomy and phacoemulsication alone in eyes with extremely shallow anterior chamber.

Materials and Methods

Patients

We studied 40 eyes of 40 Japanese patients with the anterior chamber depth equal to or less than 2.5 mm. A diagnosis of glaucoma was on the gonioscopic finding, appearance of the optic nerve head cupping and visual alteration according to the guideline of Japan Glaucoma Society. [3] Excluded were patients with post-traumatic, uveitic, neovascular, or dysgenetic glaucoma, as well as patients with eyes with greater than 25 % of peripheral anterior synechiae which needed to receive goniosynechialysis. [4-6] The study protocol and consent forms were approved by the Human Subjects Committee. Patients were informed of the purpose of our study and they provided written informed consent. The patients were prospectively randomized to receive phacoemulsication with vitrectomy or phacoemulsication alone with only one eye of a patient to be randomized. When both eyes were eligible, the right eye became the study eye. Within 24 hours after enrollment, the patients were randomized using an envelope method. In brief, we prepared each envelope which contained a card which showed either phacoemulsication with vitrectomy group or phacoemulsication alone group. Within 24 hours after enrollment, an envelope was picked-up and the inside card showed the way to treat the patient, phacoemulsication with vitrectomy or phacoemulsication alone. A total of 20 patients underwent phacoemulsication with vitrectomy and the remaining 20 patients underwent phacoemulsication alone. Treatment began within a week after these random assignments.

Surgical Procedure and Postoperative Interventions

In the phacoemulsication with vitrectomy group, sutureless transconjunctival single-port vitrectomy was carried out using 25-gauge vitreous cutter (Biological Instrumental Developmental Laboratories Inc., San Leadro, CA, USA) and 25-gauge cannula system (DORC, Zuid-Holland,

The Netherlands) prior to phacoemulsification until vitreous pressure was reduced to make the anterior chamber deep enough to facilitate the further procedure . Phacoemulsification and intraocular lens implantation was performed through a superior sclerocorneal incision after scleral cauterization. A standard phacoemulsification technique was used. In all cases, a one-piece hydrophobic acrylic intraocular lens (AcrySof™ MA30BM; Alcon, Fort Worth, TX, USA) was implanted. Sodium hyaluronate 1% (Healon, AMO, Santana, CA, USA) was used as viscoelastics.

In both groups, all patients were given topical levofloxacin and nevafenac three times daily during the first 2 weeks, tapered over the next 2 months. Nevafenac, a nonsteroidal anti-inflammatory drug, was used to reduce inflammation instead of steroid. [7].

Evaluation of Outcomes

Before enrollment, patients read and signed an Institutional Review Board–approved informed consent before any procedures were performed in this study. Patients had an ocular and systemic history taken as well as slit-lamp biomicroscopy, visual acuity and gonioscopy. The optic nerve was examined with a Goldman three-mirror lens and measurements were taken of the size of the disc, the vertical and horizontal cup/disc ratios, the presence of rim notching or splinter hemorrhage, and the presence of peripapillary atrophy. Best-corrected visual acuity and intraocular pressure was measured at every visit, and the log of the minimum angle of resolution (logMAR) was calculated and used for all statistical analyses. Goldman applanation tonometry was carried out to measure intraocular pressure. Three measurements were recorded in each eye, the mean of which was used in the calculations. Preoperative nuclear sclerosis was graded clinically at the slit lamp examination as described by Emery and Little. [8] Anterior chamber depth was measured with A-mode ultrasonography (Ultrasonic B Scanner UD-8000, Tomey, Nagoya, Japan). Measurements were repeated 10 times, the mean of which was used in the statistics. Measurement of corneal endothelial cell density was carried out with specular microscope (SP.2000, TOPCON, Tokyo, Japan).

Patient progress was reviewed at 1 and 3 days, 1 week, 1 month, 3months and 6 months after surgery. The presence of complications was determined intraoperatively and at every postoperative visit. Hypotony was defined as an intraocular pressure of less than 4 mmHg after surgery. A shallow/flat anterior chamber was defined as reported by Teehasaenee and Ritch. [9] An intraocular pressure spike was defined as an intraocular pressure on the first postoperative day of greater than or equal to 3 mmHg higher than the preoperative level.

Study End

All patients were meant to reach a 12-month follow-up, but the following were considered as endpoints: (1) the need for any further surgical procedure; (2) patient failure to attend scheduled visits, allowing for a margin of tolerance. If the study was ended before month 6, the last values obtained in the trial were considered as the final data.

Statistical Analysis

Evaluation of continuous variables was achieved using the Student's t-test. To evaluate the difference in intraocular pressures and corneal endothelial cell density between follow-up intervals, the paired t-test was used. All t-tests were two-tailed. Categoric variables were evaluated with the chi-square test, the Fisher exact test, or the Spearman rank correlation as appropriate. A level of $P < 0.05$ was accepted as statistically significant.

For the pairing of groups, the age, sex, best-corrected visual acuity, anterior chamber depth and intraocular pressure at baseline were used for matching. We studied a correlation between the paired observations. If observations were correlated, the F-test was used to study two population variances.

Results

Baseline

Patient demographics are summarized in Table 1. Mean age was 79.9 ± 6.1 years in the phacoemulsification with vitrectomy group and 80.6 ± 5.6 years in the phacoemulsification alone group (P = 0.7). No significant difference was found in age, gender, best-corrected visual acuity and intraocular pressure between the two groups. Mean anterior chamber depth was 2.19 ± 0.23 mm in the phacoemulsication with vitrectomy group and 2.17 ± 0.25 mm in the phacoemulsication alone group (P = 0.9).

Table 1. Background of the patients

	Phacoemulsification with vitrectomy group	Phacoemulsification alone group	P
Number of patients (number of eyes)	20 (20)	20 (20)	
Age (years)	79.9±6.1 (70-92)	80.6±5.6 (70-91)	0.7
Gender	15 females 5 males	13 females 7males	0.5
Anterior chamber depth (mm)	2.19±0.23 (1.73-2.48)	2.17±0.25 (1.68-2.47)	0.8
Nuclear sclerosis	3.8±0.6 (3-5)	3.9±0.6 (3-5)	0.6
Best-corrected visual acuity	0.189 (20/105.7)	0.181 (20/110.5)	
Mean (LogMAR) ± SD	0.723 ± 0.261	0.742 ± 0.260	0.8
Intraocular pressure (mmHg)	17.0±4.7 (11-26)	17.4±4.2 (13-25)	0.8
Corneal endothelial cell density (/mm^2)	2420±360 (1532 – 2878)	2436±313 (1643 – 3015)	0.9
Nd:YAG Laser iridotomy	7 (35%)	5 (25%)	0.5
Previous glaucoma attack	3 (15%)	2 (10%)	0.6
Pseudoexfoliation syndrome	2 (10%)	3 (15%)	0.6

Parenthesis indicates a range.
LogMAR ± SD: Log of the minimum angle of resolution ± Standard Deviation

Postoperative Visual Improvement and Intraocular Pressure Change

All patients were completely followed-up (Table 2). All patients in both groups showed a significant visual improvement at any postoperative visit. There was no significant difference in the mean best-corrected visual acuity between the two groups at any time point before and after surgery. Best-corrected visual acuity at baseline and at 6 months postoperatively was 0.189 and 0.756 in the phacoemulsification with vitrectomy group and 0.181 and 0.777 in the phacoemusification alone group, respectively. A change of Log MAR of best-corrected visual acuity at 6 months was -0.601 ± 0.263 in the phacoemusification with vitrectomy group and -0.633 ± 0.287 in the phacoemulsification alone group (P= 0.7) (Table 2).

Table 2. A Change of Best-corrected Visual Acuity in the phacoemulsification with vitrectomy group and the phacoemusification alone group

	Phacoemulsification with vitrectomy group	Phacoemulsification alone group	P
Number of eyes	20	20	
Baseline	0.189 (20/105.7)	0.181 (20/110.5)	
Mean (LogMAR) ± SD	0.723 ± 0.261	0.742 ± 0.260	0.8
1 month	0.799 (20/25.0)	0.768 (20/26.0)	
Mean (LogMAR) ± SD	0.098 ± 0.159	0.109 ± 0.077	0.8
Change of LogMAR	-0.625 ± 0.249	-0.628 ± 0.274	0.9
6 months	0.756 (20/26.5)	0.777 (20/25.7)	
Mean (LogMAR) ± SD	0.121 ± 0.164	0.109 ± 0.139	0.8
Change of LogMAR	-0.601 ± 0.263	-0.633 ± 0.287	0.7

Parenthesis indicates a range.

No significant difference was found in the intraocular pressure and its change between the two groups at any visit. Mean change at 6 months was -3.0±2.3 mmHg in the phacoemulsification with vitrectomy group and -3.0±2.9 mmHg in the phacoemusification alone group (P = 1.0) (Table 3). No additional anti-glaucoma surgery was necessary in the two groups.

Table 3. A change of intraocular pressure in the phacoemulsification with vitrectomy group and the phacoemusification alone group

	Phacoemulsification with vitrectomy group	Phacoemulsification alone group	P
Number of eyes	20	20	
Intraocular pressure (mmHg)			
Baseline	17.0±4.7 (11-26)	17.4±4.2 (13-25)	0.8
1 week	14.4±3.9 (10-23)	14.1± 2.6 (11-19)	0.8
1 month	14.2±3.4 (10-22)	14.0±2.0 (11-18)	0.8
3 months	14.2±3.2 (10-20)	14.1±2.3 (11-18)	0.9
6 months	14.0±2.9 (10-20)	14.5±2.3 (12-20)	0.5
Change of intraocular pressure (mmHg)			
1 week	-2.6±1.8 (-8 - 0)	-3.3±2.6 (-11 – 0)	0.3
1 month	-2.8±1.8 (-8 - -1)	-3.5±2.9 (-11 – 0)	0.4
3 months	-2.8±1.9 (-8 – 0)	-3.3±2.9 (-10 – 0)	0.8
6 months	-3.0±2.3 (-10 – 0)	-3.0±2.9 (-10 – 0)	1.0

Parenthesis indicates a range.

A Change of Corneal Endothelial Cell Density

Corneal endothelial cell density at baseline and at 6 months postoperatively was 2420±360/mm^2 and 2282± 3331/ mm^2 in the phacoemulsication with vitrectomy group and 2436±313/mm^2 and 2248±335/mm^2 in the phacoemulsication alone group, respectively (Table 4). The phacoemulsication alone group showed a loss of 6.8±2.2 % at 1 month and 7.9±3.0 % at 6 months in the change of corneal endothelium cell density, which was significantly greater than that of the phacoemusication with vitrectomy group (at 1month, P = 0.0032; at 6 months, P = 0.0057) (Table 4).

Table 4. A change of corneal endothelial cell density in the phacoemulsification with vitrectomy group and the phacoemusification alone group

	Phacoemulsification with vitrectomy group	Phacoemulsification alone group	P
Number of eyes	20	20	
Baseline (/mm^2)	2420±360 (1532 – 2878)	2436±313 (1643 – 3015)	0.9
1 month (/mm^2)	2300±320 (1481 – 2725)	2275±316 (1460 – 2895)	0.8
Change	-4.8±1.8% (-8.1% - -1.5%)	-6.8±2.2% (-11.1% - -4.0%)	0.0032
6 months (/mm^2)	2282± 333 (1450- 2730)	2248±335 (1447 – 2922)	0.7
Change	-5.7±1.5% (-8.5% - -3.0%)	-7.9±3.0% (-15.3% - -4.1%)	0.0057

Parenthesis indicates a range.

In the phacoemulsication alone group, the corneal endothelial cell density loss significantly increased in relation to the decrease of the anterior chamber depth (P = 0.0012), whereas there was no significant correlation in the phacoemulsication with vitrectomy group (Figure 1).

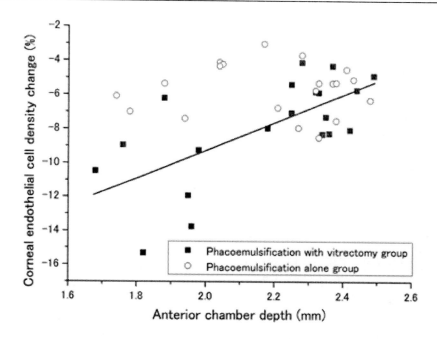

Figure 1. A relationship between anterior chamber depth and corneal endothelial cell count change in in the phacoemulsification with vitrectomy group and the phacoemusification alone group. The solid squares and solid line indicate the phacoemulsification with vitrectomy group and the open circles sindicate the phacoemulsification alone group.

Incidence of Complications and Adverse Events

Complications are listed in Table 5. No significant difference in the incidence of any complication between the phacoemulsification with vitrectomy group and the phacoemulsification alone group. Complications included two cases (10%) of continuous curvilinear capsulorhexis tear in the phacoemulsication alone group, whereas one case (5%) of zonular dehiscence occurred in each group, which led to transsscleral ciliary sulcus suture fixation of the intraocular lens.

Table 5. Incidence of intra- and postoperative complications in the phacoemulsification with vitrectomy group and the phacoemusification alone group

	Phacoemulsification with vitrectomy group	Phacoemulsification alone group	P
Number of eyes	20	20	
Intraoperative complications			
Early perforation	0 (0 %)	0 (0 %)	-
CCC tear	0 (0 %)	2 (10 %)	-
Posterior capsule rupture	0 (0 %)	0 (0 %)	0.2
Vitreous loss	0 (0 %)	0 (0 %)	-
Nucleus drop	0 (0 %)	0 (0 %)	-
Zonular dehiscence	1 (5 %)	1 (5 %)	1.0
Early postoperative complications			
Hypotony	0 (0 %)	0 (0 %)	-
IOP spike	1 (5 %)	2 (10 %)	0.4
Corneal edema	2 (10 %)	4 (20 %)	0.4
Shallow/flat anterior chamber	0 (0 %)	0 (0 %)	-
Distorted pupil	0 (0 %)	0 (0 %)	-
IOL dislocation	0 (0 %)	0 (0 %)	-
Vitreous herniation	0 (0 %)	0 (0 %)	-
Retinal detachment	0 (0 %)	0 (0 %)	-
Endophthalmitis	0 (0 %)	0 (0 %)	-

CCC tear: continuous curvilinear capsulorhexis tear.

Discussion

In the current study, there was a significant difference in postoperative loss in the corneal endothelial cell density between the phacoemulsication with 25-gauge vitrectomy group and the phacoemulsication alone group; the phacoemulsication with vitrectomy group showed 7.9 % and the phacoemulsication alone group showed 5.7 % at 6 months after surgery. In the phacoemulsication alone group, the corneal endothelial cell density loss significantly increased in relation to the decrease of the anterior chamber depth, although there was no significant correlation in the phacoemulsication with vitrectomy group. In the phacoemulsication alone group, four of seven eyes with 2.0 mm or less of preoperative anterior chamber depth showed greater than 10 % of postoperative loss although there was one eye showing the same amount of cell loss in the phacoemusification with vitrectomy group, which experienced zonular disherence and underwent transcleral ciliary sulcus fixation of the intraocular lens. There was no significant difference between the two groups in visual improvement and intraocular change. Therefore, these lines of evidence suggest that transconjunctival sutureless vitrectomy prior to phacoemulsification should be used in eyes with extremely shallow anterior chamber depth, especially those with 2.0 mm or less of the anterior chamber depth.

Although there was no significant difference noted in the incidence of intra- and postoperative complications, two eyes in the phacoemulsification alone group experienced continuous curvilinear capsulorhexis tear, whereas none in the phacoemulsification with vitrectomy group did. There was a possibility that extremely shallow anterior chamber may make the maneuver difficult and lead to the tear. The vitrectomy prior to phacoemulsificatiion can reduce the possibility of the complication.

Recent studies showed the superiority of primary phacoemulsification to laser peripheral iridotomy in the management of acute angle closure. [10,11] Husain et al. demonstrated that phacoemulsification resulted in lower rate of intraocular pressure failure at 2 years compared with laser peripheral iridotmy. [12] Park et al. showed that early phacoemulsification showed lower endothelial cell loss compared with laser iridotomy in the treatment of acute angle closure after a 2-year follow-up. [13]

This study has important limitations. The sample size of this study was small, therefore not powered to detect small differences. Small sample size also precluded assessment of safety. Futhermore, a masked study design could have reduced observer bias.

Although the sample size in each group was small, the current study demonstrated that (1) There was no significant postoperative visual improvement in between the phacoemulsication with vitrectomy group and the phacoemulsication alone group; (2) transconjunctival vitrectomy prior to phacoemulsication may reduce corneal endothelial cell loss compared with phacoemulsication alone. Future study of a large population is needed to verify these observations. However, this information may be clinically valuable when treating patients with cataract and extremely shallow anterior chamber.

Conclusion

There was no significant postoperative visual improvement in between the phacoemulsication with vitrectomy group and the phacoemulsication alone group. Phacoemulsication with vitrectomy may reduce corneal endothelial cell density loss compared with phacoemulsication alone.

References

[1] Miura S, Ieki Y, Ogino K, Tanaka Y. Primary phacoemulsification and aspiration combined with 25-gauge single-port vitrectomy for management of acute angle closure. *Eur J Ophthalmol.* 2008;18:450-2.
[2] Dada T, KImar S, Gadia R, et al. Sutureless single-port transconjunctival pars plana limited vitrectomy combined with phacoemulsification for management of phacomorphic glaucoma. *J Cataract Refract Surg.* 2007;33:951-4.
[3] The Japan Glaucoma Society guidelines of glaucoma (2nd edition). *Nippon Ganka Gakkai Zasshi.* 2006;110:777-815.
[4] Teekhasaenee C, Ritch R. Combined phacoemulsification and goniosynechialysis for uncontrolled chronic angle-closure glaucoma after acute angle-closure glaucoma. *Ophthalmology.* 1999;106:669-74.
[5] Harasymowycz PJ, Papamatheakis DG, Ahmed I, et al. Phacoemulsification and goniosynechialysis in the management of unresponsive primary angle closure. *J Glaucoma.* 2005;14:186-9.
[6] Qing G, Wang N, Mu D. Efficacy of goniosynechialysis for advanced chronic angle-closure glaucoma. *Clin Ophthalmol.* 2012;6:1723-9.
[7] Miyake K, Ibaraki N. Prostaglandins and cystoid macular edema. *Surv Ophthalmol* 2002;47(suppl 1):s203-230.
[8] Emery JM, Little HY. Phacoemulsification and aspiration of cataract: Surgical techniques, complications and results. CY Mosby, St Louis, pp45-48, 1979.
[9] Teehasaenee C, Ritch R. The use of PhEA 34c in trabeculectomy. Ophthalmology 1986;93:487-490.
[10] Lam DS, Tham CC, Lai JS, Leung DY. Current approaches to the management of acute primary angle closure. *Curr Opin Ophthalmol.* 2007;18:146-51.

[11] Boey PY, Singhal S, Perera SA, Aung T. Conventional and emerging treatments in the management of acute primary angle closure. *Clin Ophthalmol.* 2012;6:417-24.

[12] Husain R, Gazzard G, Aung T, et al. Initial management of acute primary angle closure: a randomized trial comparing phacoemulsification with laser peripheral iridotomy. *Ophthalmology.* 2012;119:2274-81.

[13] Park HY, Lee NY, Park CK, Kim MS. Long-term changes in endothelial cell counts after early phacoemulsification versus laser peripheral iridotomy using sequential argon:YAG laser technique in acute primary angle closure. *Graefes Arch Clin Exp Ophthalmol.* 2012;250:1673-80.

In: Cataracts and Cataract Surgery
Editor: Didier Navarro

ISBN: 978-1-62808-400-9
© 2013 Nova Science Publishers, Inc.

Chapter V

Teaching and Learning Cataract Surgery

Sandra M. Johnson[1],* and Eric Areiter[2]
[1]Ophthalmology University of Virginia Department of Ophthalmology
[2]University of Virginia School of Medicine

Abstract

Introduction: The most common procedure done by ophthalmology resident surgeons is cataract surgery. This is the back bone procedure for their training and aims at treating the most common cause of blindness in the world.

Methods: This chapter is based on a literature review of resident cataract surgery and resident surgery in general.

Results: Information is available on teaching the phacoemulsification techniques of cataract surgery and regarding resident outcomes for this.

Conclusion: An awareness of the methods, issues and outcomes for resident cataract surgeons can serve to enhance the practice. More information is needed regarding teaching the technique of small incision extra capsular cataract surgery.

---

* Corresponding author: smjeyes@gmail.com.

Introduction

Cataracts surgeries are among the most common operations performed by resident ophthalmologists, and have been an essential part of postgraduate education in ophthalmology for the past twenty years. Indeed, cataract is the leading cause of blindness in the world [1]. Over the course of their education, a resident in the United States will typically perform hundreds of such operations, with many of these performed at a Veterans Administration (VA) medical center. Outside of the Western nations, manual small incision cataract surgery (MSICS) is the technique that is preferred, due to its lower costs and less dependence on technology [2,3,4]. In Western nations, cataract surgery by phacoemulsification is the dominant technique taught.

However, there is a large amount of variation in United States (US) residencies as to how many cases residents actually perform, and many programs only allow third year residents to perform phacoemulsification. In 2002, the median number of cataract surgeries by phacoemulsification performed by US ophthalmology residents was 100, however at that time 13% of residents completed fewer than 70 cataract surgeries, during their three years of residency. There was a range in cataract procedures from 50 to 300 operations. Some US residency programs are seeing a decrease in volume of patients suitable for cataract surgery performed by resident ophthalmologists. One reason for this is a continually decreasing VA population and the increase in private practices lead by faculty at many universities compared to resident run clinics [5]. On the other hand, the number of cataract procedures actually performed by resident surgeons in the last several years has overall increased, due to programs ensuring they meet ACGME (Accreditation Council for Graduate Medical Education) requirements.

Training: General

There is no exact consensus on what constitutes the best program of learning for a cataract surgeon. Most programs include programmatic reading such as the lens book in the Basic Science Series for residents published by the American Academy of Ophthalmology (AAO) and major text books on cataract surgery. Journals such as the Journal of Cataract and Refractive Surgery have more advanced reading on the topic of cataract surgery. Didactic lectures are also part of the foundation for the developing surgeon, as well as the exercise of watching surgical videos and assisting more senior surgeons.

Experiential procedure-based learning during residency is especially important in ophthalmology training programs, contrasted with didactic, lecture-focused teaching. Due to the complex microsurgical procedures the field entails, simply reading about a particular procedure is insufficient to becoming proficient at it. A beginning resident surgeon can only master techniques through practice. Similarly to learning to ride a bike, reading about the process of how to best ride a bike can only take a person so far.

Surgical simulators as well as eye-bank and animal eyes are utilized by residency programs to prepare residents for phacoemulsification on patients as a primary surgeon.

Training: Wet Labs

Eye-bank and animal eyes offer residents the ability to work on actual eyes instead of only simulator work. The residency review committee (RRC) in ophthalmology in the United States has mandated that wet-lab experience is necessary for ophthalmology programs to address the practical and ethical issues raised by only live surgical training [6]. Due to the financial requirements posed on a program for simulator usage, wet-lab eyes are still one of the only ways many residents can gain cataract surgery experience prior to operating themselves. Due to ACGME requirements regarding resident teaching, evaluation, and work hours, teaching programs are incurring additional costs resulting in difficulties obtaining expensive simulators [5].

Differences between animal eyes and human ones pose some difficulties in resident training, though they are anatomically quite similar. The porcine lens capsule being very elastic and tense has been found to make capsulorhexis more difficult to perform than in actual human patients, and in a post-mortem wet lab setting the porcine cornea becomes less transparent. Porcine lenses are also large and soft, and porcine specimens have larger anterior chambers than human specimens. Vacuum phacoemulsification for nucleus quadrant removal on human patients in the operating room requires both coordination of hands and feet. While coordination of hands and feet is necessary in a surgical simulator, in the wet-lab using eye-bank and animal eyes it may not be. However, wet-lab practice has improved over time, with advances such as cataract induction, animal eye preparation, and globe-positioning devices, increasing the wet lab usefulness to new surgeons [7]. While human eyes in the wet-lab are preferable to porcine ones, it is difficult to obtain specimens with well-developed cataracts and a clear cornea for resident surgeons to operate on. Artificially manufactured eyes can be employed for practicing particular steps of cataracts surgery such as nucleus removal, though differences between artificial and live specimens make training with them difficult. The Kitaro wet and dry lab systems is one such product that can be useful for learning particular steps such as capsulorhexis (FCI Ophthalmics, Marshfield, MA, USA).

To assess competency in ophthalmologic surgical skills, the wet-lab based Eye Surgical Skills Assessment Test (ESSAT) is employed by resident programs throughout the US. This exam consists of evaluation in the areas of skin suturing, muscle recession, and phacoemulsification, and residents are evaluated either live or by video according to a task-specific checklist with a global rating scale [8]. ESSAT usage, prior to entering the operating room as a primary surgeon, ensures that residents have a basic level of competency to ensure lower morbidity of their patients early in their surgical training.

Training: Simulators

Surgical simulators offer residents the opportunity to practice particular techniques extensively and result in decreased morbidity in their future patients. The curvilinear capsulorhexis technique performed during cataract extraction has been found to be challenging for new surgeons to perform well, and the Eyesi surgery simulator can be used to master this [9]. It has been found to improve resident surgical skills, including superior wet-lab capsulorhexis performed in residents after structured training with Eyesi [10]. It has been found that residents who trained with surgical simulators prior to perfomring surgery on human patients had shorter durations of total phacoemulsification time, used a lower intraoperative phaco power, and had fewer intraoperative complications early on in their surgical training [11].

Training: Operating Room

The survey of ophthalmic surgical trainees performed in the United Kingdom found that trainees had dissatisfaction with surgical training in the areas of attitudes and skill of trainers, poor structure of training rotations, and insufficient opportunities to practice surgical procedures both in the operating room and in the wet-lab. To maximize operating room training, the techniques of modular training, reverse training, and sequential training are employed

[12,13]. Modular training gives a resident surgeon the opportunity to perform a particular part of an operation on cases, with residents becoming well trained in one technique of a procedure in a relatively short amount of time. Reverse training is a widely used practice giving the training surgeon instruction on learning a procedure in reverse order. This can be useful in phacoemulsification training; due to the greater technical proficiency needed for earlier steps compared to later ones. Sequential training gives a resident surgeon a specified amount of time in which to perform a procedure, after which an attending physician takes over as the primary surgeon. This can be useful in busy facilities to prevent the daily schedule of patients from becoming too backed up, due to an inexperienced resident taking an extensive amount of time performing aspects of a procedure. In the United Kingdom national cataract training survey, trainers have been found to prefer modular training over reverse training, and the least preferred method has been found to be sequential training [12]. One system of sequential training is the Zwisch proposed model for teaching. It uses an assessment that describes a continuum from first assisting as an observer through recovering one's own errors, working with an inexperienced first assistant and knowing when to seek advice [14].

Outcomes

It has been established, in general surgery, that cases performed by residents result in patients' who experience a higher postsurgical morbidity and mortality. This correlates with surgeries performed with less experienced residents at the beginning of a new academic year [15]. Cataract extraction by phacoemulsification with resident participation has significantly increased operating times when the resident is in the first half of their academic year [16], and some studies have found surgical complication rates of third-year residents performing phacoemulsification to be higher than what is reported by attending ophthalmologists [17]. In particular, after 80 cases have been performed by a particular resident, a significant reduction has been found in vitreous loss and mean adjusted time for total phacoemulsification procedure [18]. Thus, in 2007, the ACGME increased the requirement of resident-performed cataracts surgeries, in which the resident is the primary surgeon, from 45 to 86 [19].

When overall complication rates of phacoemulsification performed by second and third year residents is examined, no significant difference has been found [5]. However, this may partially be attributable to cases being assigned to second year residents with fewer risk factors than what may be given to a third year. Regarding individual complications, wound burns have been seen more frequently in phacoemulsification performed by third year residents, while capsule tears were seen more often in procedures performed by second year residents. Vitreous loss has been found to be more common in cataracts surgeries performed by second year residents, though there is no consensus in the literature regarding this[20]. There is little overall consensus in the literature regarding complication trends and long term outcomes when comparing resident-performed surgical cases with more experienced surgeons [6].

Conclusion

Training cataract surgeons is an important task given the global burden of this condition and the importance of good vision in the quality of life. Awareness of the ways in which this is taught and research and publication of novel teaching techniques in this area should contribute to better outcomes. More data needs to be collected on teaching of small incision extra capsular techniques which are the mainstay of cataract procedures in many countries.

References

[1] Rao, GN; Khanna, R; Payal, A. The global burden of cataract. *Curr Opn Ophthal*, 2010; 22, 4-9.
[2] Khanna, RC; Kaza, S; Palamaner, SSG; Shantha, G; et al. Comparative outcomes of manual small incision cataract surgery and phacoemulsification performed by ophthalmology trainees in a tertiary eye care hospital in India: a retrospective cohort design. *BMJ Open*, 2012; 2:e001035. doi:10.1136/bmjopen-2012-001035.
[3] DeCroos, FC; Chow, JH; Garg, P; et al. Analysis of resident performed manual small incision cataract surgery (MSICS): an efficacious approach to mature cataracts. *Int Ophthal*. 2012; 32, 547-52.
[4] Jongsareejit, A; Wiriyaluppa, C; Kongsap, P; Phumipan, S. Cost effectiveness analysis of manual small incision cataract surgery

(MSICS) and phacoemulsification (PE). *J Med Assoc Thai*, 2012; 95, 212-20.

[5] Smith, JS. Teaching phacoemulsification in US ophthalmology residencies: can the quality be maintained? *Curr Opin Ophthalmol*, 2005; 16, 27–32.

[6] Lee, A; Greenlee, E; Oetting, T; Beaver, H; Johnson, T; Boldt, H; Abramoff, M; Olson, R; Carter, K. The Iowa Ophthalmology Wet Laboratory Curriculum for Teaching and Assessing Cataract Surgical Competency. *Ophthalmology*, 2007; 114, e21–e26

[7] Henderson, B; Grimes, K; Fintelmann, R; Oetting, T. Stepwise approach to establishing an ophthalmology wet laboratory. *J Cataract Refract Surg*, 2009; 35, 1121–1128.

[8] Taylor, JB; Binenbaum, G; Tapino, P; Volpe, NJ. Microsurgical lab testing is a reliable method for assessing ophthalmology residents' surgical skills. *Br J Ophthalmol*, 2007; 91, 1691–1694.

[9] Webster, R; Sassani, J; Shenk, R; Harris, M; Gerber, J; Benson, A; Blumenstock, J; Billman, C; Haluck, R. Simulating the curvilinear capsulorhexis procedure during cataract surgery on the EYESi system *Stud Health Technol Inform*, 111 (2005), 592–595.

[10] Feudner, EM; Engel, C; Neuhann, IM; Petermeier, K; Bartz-Schmidt, K-U; Szurman, P. Virtual reality training improves wet-lab performance of capsulorhexis: results of a randomized, controlled study *Graefes Arch Clin Exp Ophthalmol*, 247 (2009), 955–963.

[11] Belyea, DA; Brown, SE; Rajjoub, LZ. Influence of surgery simulator training on ophthalmology resident phacoemulsification performance. *J Cataract Refract Surg.* 2011 Oct; 37(10), 1756-61. doi: 10.1016/j.jcrs.2011.04.032. Epub 2011 Aug 15.

[12] Alexander, P; Matheson, D; Baxter, J; Tint, N. United Kingdom national cataract training survey. *J Cataract Refract Surg*, 2012; 38, 533–538.

[13] Benjamin, L. Training in Surgical Skills. *Commun Eye Health*, 2002; 15(42), 19–20.

[14] DeRosa, DA; Zwischenberger, JB; Meyerson, SL; et al. A theory-based model for teaching and assessing residents in the operating room. *J Surg Educ*, 2013; 70, 24-30.

[15] Englesbe, MJ; Pelletier, SJ; Magee, JC; Magee, JC; Gauger, P; Schifftner, T; Henderson, WG; Khuri, SF; Campbell, DA. Seasonal variation in surgical outcomes as measured by the American College of Surgeons-National Surgical Quality Improvement Program (ACS-NSQIP). *Ann Surg.* 2007 Sep; 246(3), 456-62; discussion 463-5.

[16] Hosler, MR; Scott, IU; Kunselman, AR; Wolford, KR; Oltra, EZ; Murray, WB. Impact of resident participation in cataract surgery on operative time and cost. *Ophthalmology*. 2012 Jan; 119(1), 95-8.

[17] Bhagat, N; Nissirios, N; Potdevin, L; Chung, J; Lama, P; Zarbin, MA; Fechtner, R; Guo, S; Chu, D; Langer, P. Complications in resident-performed phacoemulsification cataract surgery at New Jersey Medical School. *Br J Ophthalmology*. 2007 Oct; 91(10), 1315-7.

[18] Randleman, JB; Wolfe, JD; Woodward, M; Lynn, MJ; Cherwek, DH; Srivastava, SK. The resident surgeon phacoemulsification learning curve *Arch Ophthalmol*, 125 (2007), 1215–1219.

[19] Accreditation Council for Graduate Medical Education. Ophthalmology resident operative minimum requirements. OPH_A A_4.5.2010. A vailable at: http://www.acgme.org/acWebsite/RRC_240/240_Minimums OperativeTable.pdf. Accessed July 24, 2009.

[20] Lee, JS; Hou, CH; Yang, ML; et al. A different approach to assess resident phacoemulsification learning curve: analysis of both completion and complication rates. *Eye* (Lond), 2009; 23, 683–7.

[21] Woodfield, Alonzo S; Gower, Emily W; Cassard, Sandra D; Saraswathy Ramanthan. Intraoperative phacoemulsification complication rates of second- and third-year ophthalmology residents a 5-year comparison. *Ophthalmology*. 2011; 18(5), 954-958.

[22] Gibson, A; Boulton, MG; Watson, MP; Moseley, MJ; Murray, PI; Fielder, AR. The first cut is the deepest: basic surgical training in ophthalmology. *Eye* 2005; 19, 1264–1270.

In: Cataracts and Cataract Surgery
Editor: Didier Navarro

ISBN: 978-1-62808-400-9
© 2013 Nova Science Publishers, Inc.

Chapter VI

Phacolytic Glaucoma

Kayoung Yi[1] and Teresa C. Chen[2]
[1]Department of Ophthalmology, Kangnam Sacred Heart Hospital,
College of Medicine, Hallym University, Seoul, Korea.
[2]Harvard Medical School, Boston, Massachusetts,
Department of Ophthalmology, Glaucoma Service,
Massachusetts Eye and Ear Infirmary,
Boston, Massachusetts, US

Abstract

Phacolytic glaucoma is a rare complication of an advanced cataract. Phacolytic glaucoma is usually an acute open angle glaucoma that develops from blockade of the trabecular meshwork by leakage of lens protein from a mature or hypermature cataract. Even though the incidence of phacolytic glaucoma is decreasing due to the availability of earlier cataract surgery, it is still in the differential diagnosis of acute elevated intraocular pressure (IOP) in patients with a dense cataract. Although phacolytic glaucoma usually occurs with a mature or hypermature cataract, it less is associated with focal liquefaction of an immature cataract. Slit lamp examination reveals high eye pressures with corneal edema, mid-dilated pupil, intense flare and large cells, and/or hyperrefringent particles. Keratic precipitates are not typically present. Initial treatment is focused on lowering the IOP with glaucoma medications and decreasing the inflammation with topical steroids. Definitive treatment is cataract extraction. The prognosis of phacolytic glaucoma is usually excellent, but delayed treatment may cause permanent damage to the optic nerve and/or cornea, resulting in a poor outcome. If IOP elevation persists after cataract surgery, additional medical and/or surgical management may be required.

Introduction

Phacolytic glaucoma (PG), a rare complication of cataract, is the sudden onset of open-angle glaucoma caused by a leaking mature or hypermature cataract. [1, 2, 3] PG is infrequent in developed countries such as the United States due to earlier cataract surgery and/ or better access to health care. However, it is still in the differential diagnosis of acute elevated intraocular pressure (IOP) in patients with advanced cataracts, especially in underdeveloped countries [4].

Clinical Presentation

PG typically occurs in the older population.[5] Patients typically present with sudden onset of a red and painful eye with a history of gradual decline in visual acuity reflecting maturation of a cataract (Figure 1). Examination reveals high IOP, microcystic corneal edema, heavy flare, aqueous cells which are thought to be macrophages (larger than the lymphocytes in uveitis), and a mature or hypermature cataract. Aggregates of white material and iridescent or hyperrefringent particles can be also detected. The latter represent calcium oxalate and cholesterol crystals being liberated from the degenerating cataractous lens (Figure 2). [6] Unlike uveitic glaucoma (such as that seen in phacoanaphylactic glaucoma), no keratic precipitates typically are present [7, 8]. Gonioscopy reveals an open anterior chamber angle. [3-9]. Usually, the fellow eye also has a cataract and a deep anterior chamber [5].

A mature cataract (totally opacified), hypermature cataract (liquid cortex and free-floating nucleus), and focal liquefaction of an immature cataract as well as a dislocated cataractous lens in the vitreous all can cause PG. [5, 10].

Pathophysiology

PG is an acute open-angle glaucoma resulted from the leakage of lens material from a dense cataract (especially a hypermature or Morgagnian cataract) through an intact lens capsule. [5] The cells in the anterior chamber of PG patients are thought to be macrophages swollen with eosinophilic lenticular material that have been ingested (Figure 3). [5]

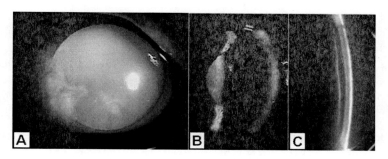

Figure 1. Anterior segment photographs of a 65-year old male who visited the emergency room for left eye pain and vomiting. He had bare hand motions vision in his left eye. The IOP of the left eye was 69mmHg. A; Slit lamp exam revealed a hypermature cataract and a pterygium. The pupil reacted sluggishly. B; A deep anterior chamber contains proteinous material and large cells. C; The van Herick method reveals a deep peripheral anterior chamber angle. Phacolytic glaucoma was diagnosed. After cataract extraction and thorough irrigation of the anterior chamber, the IOP was normalized without long-term complications. (Courtesy of Dr Shin Hee Kang).

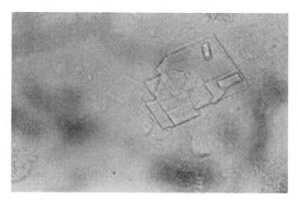

Figure 2. Microscopy of the aspirate at the time of cataract extraction shows clumped, notched rectangular platelike crystals from the aqueous of a patient with phacolytic glaucoma (X160). Reproduced from *J Korean Ophthalmol Soc* 2000 Sep;41(9): Copyright © 2000, Korean Ophthalmological Society. All rights reserved.

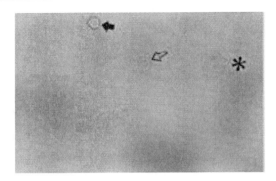

Figure 3. Microscopy of the aspirate at the time of cataract extraction of a patient with phacolytic glaucoma shows round, regular cells with foamy cytoplasm consistent with macrophages (*). A leukocyte (white arrow) and an erythrocyte (black arrow) also are seen (X160). Reproduced from J Korean Ophthalmol Soc 2000 Sep;41(9): Copyright © 2000, Korean Ophthalmological Society. All rights reserved.

Originally these macrophages were thought to be the cause of blockade of the trabecular meshwork (TM), but the heavy molecular weight (HMW) lens protein leaking from the intact capsule is regarded to play a more significant role in obstructing the TM. [5, 9, 11, 12]. The typical macrophage response is believed to be a natural response to lens protein in the anterior chamber rather than the cause of the outflow obstruction [5].

In a recent report, the possibility of two forms of PG was proposed; a hyperacute presentation caused by rapid leakage of degenerated lens proteins which block the TM and a second type with a more gradual onset and with macrophages in the anterior chamber resulting from an immunologic response to leaking lens proteins [9, 13].

Diagnosis

A typical history and clinical presentation may be enough to make a diagnosis of PG. In their study on PG, Mandal and Gothwal made the diagnosis of PG based on the following signs and symptoms: 1) a history of progressive visual loss followed by acute onset of pain, redness, and epiphora; 2) high IOP with or without corneal edema; 3) presence of circulating small chunks of white material with variable content of cells and flare; 4) occasional pseudohypopyon in the anterior chamber without keratic precipitates; 5) presence of a mature or a hypermature cataract with white capsular patches; 6) no evidence of trauma; and 7) a deep anterior chamber with a gonioscopically open angle [8]. In questionable cases, a diagnostic paracentesis can reveal characteristic swollen macrophages with engulfed lens material (Figure 2) [6].

Treatment

Even though the definitive treatment is the removal of cataract, initial medical treatment is necessary to lower the IOP and control the pain and discomfort. [5]

Patients with phacolytic glaucoma can be managed with topical cycloplegia, topical steroids, and aqueous suppressants initially. [5] If the IOP is severely elevated or does not respond to initial topical medications, a systemic carbonic anhydrase inhibitor and an osmotic agent may be considered.

The definitive treatment of PG is cataract extraction. Extracapsular cataract extraction (ECCE) with an intraocular lens implant is considered the treatment of choice. [4, 8, 14, 15] Using a dye such as trypan blue during capsulotomy may be needed for better visualization of the anterior capsule in a mature or hypermature cataract. [4, 15] Poor visual potential is not a contraindication for surgery [8]

IOP begins to normalize following cataract extraction, allowing discontinuation of IOP lowering treatment in most cases. A minority of patients with persistent elevation of IOP may need long-term medical therapy or a filtering surgery to control IOP [14].

Prognosis is often excellent, with marked improvement in vision in many patients following cataract extraction; however, delayed treatment may cause a poor outcome. [14-16] Patients with phacolytic glaucoma (PG) may have a worse prognosis than patients with phacomorphic glaucoma. [14, 16] Subluxation of the lens and postoperative inflammation were more severe in phacolytic glaucoma compared to other lens-induced glaucomas. [16] Uncontrolled glaucoma and/or persistent corneal edema can be responsible for loss of vision. Other surgical complications, including suprachoroidal hemorrhage, capsular rupture with loss of lens material into the posterior segment, corneal injury, and vitreous prolapse also can happen. [15] Vitreous opacification behind the posterior capsule due to the accumulation of lens protein released through the microleaks in the posterior capsule is a unique phenomenon of PG [8].

Conclusion

PG is a complication of an advanced cataract and presents as an acute open-angle glaucoma. The typical clinical signs include a mature or hypermature cataract and a deep anterior chamber with large cells and/or proteinous lens material with a grossly intact lens capsule. The majority of patients can be initially managed medically, but definitive management usually requires surgical removal of the cataract [2, 3, 5].

References

[1] Kanski JJ. Lens-related glaucoma. In: *Clinical Ophthalmology*. 6th ed. Butterworth Heinemann; 2007:408-410.
[2] Richter C. Lens-induced open angle glaucoma: phacolytic glaucoma (lens protein glaucoma). In: Ritch R, Shields MB, Krupin T, eds. *The Glaucomas*. 2nd ed. St Louis: Mosby; 1996:1023-1026.
[3] Shaarawy TM, Sherwood MB, Hitchings RA, Crowston JG. Other Secondary glaucomas. In: *Glaucoma*.; Saunders Elsevier; 2009:419.
[4] Venkatesh R, Tan CS, Kumar TT, Ravindran RD. Safety and efficacy of manual small incision cataract surgery for phacolytic glaucoma. *Br. J. Ophthalmol*. 2007;91(3):279-81.
[5] Papaconstantinou D, Georgalas I, Kourtis N, Krassas A, Diagourtas A, Koutsandrea C, Georgopoulos G. Lens-induced glaucoma in the elderly. *Clin. Interv. Aging*. 2009;4:331-6.
[6] Kim IT, Jung BY, Shim JY. Cholesterol crystals in aqueous humor of the eye with phacolytic glaucoma. *J. Korean Ophthalmol. Soc.* 2000;41(9):2003-7.
[7] Allingham RR, Damji KD, Freedman S. Glaucomas associated with disorders of the lens: phacolytic (lens protein) glaucoma. In: *Shields Textbook of Glaucoma*. 2005. 5th ed. Philadelphia: Lippincott Williams and Wilkins; 262-3.
[8] Mandal AK, Gothwal VK. Intraocular pressure control and visual outcome in patients with phacolytic glaucoma managed by extracapsular cataract extraction with or without posterior chamber intraocular lens implantation. *Ophthalmic. Surg. Lasers*. Nov 1998;29(11):880-9.

[9] Mavrakanas N, Axmann S, Issum CV, Schutz JS, Shaarawy T. Phacolytic Glaucoma: Are There 2 Forms?. *J. Glaucoma.* 2012; 21(4):248-9.
[10] Chu ER, Durkin SR, Keembiyage RD, Nathan F, Raymond G. Nineteen-year delayed-onset phacolytic uveitis following dislocation of the crystalline lens. *Can. J. Ophthalmol.* Feb 2009;44(1):112.
[11] Epstein DL, Jedziniak J, Grant WM. Identification of heavy molecular weight soluble protein in aqueous humor in human phacolytic glaucoma. *Invest. Ophthalmol. Vis. Sci.* 1978;17:398–402.
[12] Feder RS, Dueker DK. Can macrophage cause obstruction to aqueous outflow in rabbits? *Int. ophthalmol.* 1984;7:87-93.
[13] Khandelwal R. Ocular snow storm: an unusual presentation of phacolytic glaucoma. BMJ Case Reports 2012;10.1136/bcr-2012-006330.
[14] Braganza A, Thomas R, George T. Management of phacolytic glaucoma: experience of 135 cases. *Indian J. Ophthalmol.* Sep 1998; 46(3):139-43.
[15] Tabin G. Safety and efficacy of manual small incision cataract surgery for phacolytic glaucoma. Br J Ophthalmol. 2007;91(3):269-70.
[16] Pradhan D, Hennig A, Kumar J. A prospective study of 413 cases of lens-induced glaucoma in Nepal. *Indian J. Ophthalmol.* 2001; Jun;49(2):103-7.

Index

A

access, 146
accommodation, 11, 13, 15, 16, 17, 23, 33, 64, 65, 77, 79
acid, 67
adaptability, 29
adaptation, 18
adhesions, 74
adults, 4, 62, 101, 104
aetiology, 101
Africa, 60
age, 13, 60, 61, 62, 66, 77, 78, 79, 83, 84, 87, 89, 90, 91, 92, 93, 94, 98, 100, 101, 102, 103, 104, 106, 107, 108, 109, 113, 127
aggregation, 91, 97
agonist, 115, 116
albumin, 93
alcohol consumption, 95
alcoholism, 64, 95
algorithm, 25, 31
allele, 74, 75
alternative medicine, viii, 111, 112
amblyopia, 77
amino, 78, 82
amino acid, 78, 82
amplitude, 13, 15, 17, 79
anatomy, vii, 1, 2
anhydrase, 149

aniridia, 71, 75, 76
ANOVA, 13
anterior chamber, vii, viii, 2, 16, 20, 23, 65, 71, 72, 74, 76, 77, 83, 84, 85, 86, 98, 114, 116, 117, 118, 124, 125, 126, 127, 130, 131, 132, 133, 139, 146, 147, 148, 150
anti-glaucoma, 129
antioxidant, 91, 95, 97
apoptosis, 107
aqueous humor, 79, 93, 150, 151
Argentina, 60
argon, 135
ARs, 113, 114
arterial hypertension, 114
arteritis, 86
artery, 74, 79
arthritis, 99
Artisan, 56
ascorbic acid, 108
aspirate, 147, 148
aspiration, 116, 134
assessment, 4, 13, 16, 21, 133, 141
asthma, 84
astigmatism, 65, 76
asymmetry, 77
atmosphere, 93
atopic dermatitis, 84, 99
atrophy, 84, 86, 99, 126
attitudes, 140

Index

autosomal dominant, 61, 71, 72, 76, 81, 105
autosomal recessive, 61, 75, 77, 78, 80
awareness, ix, 90, 137

B

Barbados, 90, 91, 95, 102, 104, 105
basement membrane, 68, 83
behaviors, 97
Beijing, 109
benign, 113, 120
benign prostatic hyperplasia, 113, 120
bias, 133
bilateral, 41, 51, 54, 56
billowing, viii, 111, 112, 115
biocompatibility, 43
births, 61
blindness, vii, ix, 59, 60, 61, 100, 103, 105, 109, 137, 138
blood, 21, 33, 79, 106
blood vessels, 21, 33, 106
body mass index, 98, 103
bone, ix, 137
breakdown, 92

C

cadmium, 95, 101, 106
calcium, 62, 91, 97, 146
calibration, 16
calorie, 98
capsule, 20, 30, 64, 65, 66, 68, 69, 71, 72, 73, 74, 80, 81, 82, 84, 85, 89, 98, 99, 114, 117, 132, 139, 142, 147, 148, 149, 150
carotene, 94, 100
carotenoids, 94
cataract extraction, ix, 85, 86, 120, 140, 145, 147, 148, 149, 150
cauterization, 126
cell cycle, 97
central obesity, 104
chaperones, 97
chemical(s), 65, 67, 108

chemosis, 85
Chicago, 23
childhood, 61, 77, 89, 100, 102
children, 4, 69, 77, 82
China, 60
cholesterol, 81, 146
chromosome, 76, 82, 102
cigarette smoke, 95, 106
cigarette smokers, 106
cigarette smoking, 100, 101
city, 100
clarity, 10, 79
classes, 69
classification, 87
cleavage, 62
climates, 67
clinical assessment, 33
clinical presentation, 85, 112, 148
closure, 75, 76, 86, 133, 134, 135
clustering, 102
clusters, 97
coenzyme, 70, 78
coherence, 16
color, 62, 63
coma, 7, 22
commercial, 123
community, 33, 102
compensation, 21, 24
complexity, vii, 1, 2, 10
compliance, 16
complications, vii, viii, 76, 77, 85, 111, 121, 124, 126, 132, 133, 134, 140, 142, 147, 149
compounds, 67
comprehension, 10
compression, 62, 65
computation, 18
computer, 4, 24
conduction, 81
configuration, 69, 71
congenital cataract, 61, 70, 71, 82, 105, 108
conjunctiva, 67
consensus, 13, 138, 142
consent, 125
construction, 116

Index   155

consulting, 4
consumption, 95
contour, 4, 10, 23
contrast sensitivity, 7, 8, 9, 33
controversial, 67
contusion, 65
cooking, 29, 93, 94, 106
coordination, 139
copper, 68, 80, 95, 101
copyright, 147, 148
cornea, ix, 22, 24, 66, 67, 74, 75, 81, 84, 85, 86, 120, 139, 146
corneal edema, ix, 117, 145, 146, 148, 149
corneal endothelium, viii, 124, 130
correlation(s), 20, 26, 30, 31, 127, 130, 132
cortex, 63, 64, 66, 68, 71, 72, 79, 80, 81, 85, 86, 88, 146
corticosteroid therapy, 82, 83
corticosteroids, 68, 85, 104
cost, 144
crown, 72
crystalline, 11, 16, 22, 23, 84, 151
crystals, 81, 146, 147, 150
CSF, 8
cycles, 7, 19
cycloplegia, 149
cysteine, 77
cystoid macular edema, 114, 134
cytokines, 109
cytomegalovirus, 82
cytoplasm, 62, 148

D

damages, 99
data collection, 32
decay, 10
defects, 80, 81
defense mechanisms, 91, 92
deficiency(s), 76, 77, 80, 94
deformation, 73
dehiscence, ix, 114, 124, 131, 132
dehydration, 94, 98
Democratic Republic of Congo, 59
Denmark, 60, 111

density values, 30
deposition, 67, 68, 69, 81, 84
deposits, 68, 69, 82, 84
depth, viii, 2, 14, 16, 29, 33, 124, 125, 126, 127, 128, 130, 131, 132
depth perception, 29
dermatitis, 84
destruction, 80
detachment, 132
detection, 64
developed countries, 146
diabetes, 79, 91, 95, 98, 104
diabetic cataract, 79, 108
diabetic patients, 79, 96
diabetic retinopathy, 5, 104
diarrhea, 94, 98
diet, 78, 80, 92, 93, 95
differential diagnosis, ix, 145, 146
diffraction, 18
dilation, 18, 77, 114, 117, 118, 119, 120
diplopia, 29, 63, 64, 65, 76
direct measure, 16
disability, 7, 8, 23, 73, 77, 78, 81
discomfort, 149
discrimination, 29, 63
diseases, 26, 27, 29, 70, 91, 96, 99, 103, 107, 108, 113
dislocated lens, 78
dislocation, 65, 77, 105, 132, 151
disorder, 76, 77, 78, 80, 81, 84
displacement, 75, 76
dissatisfaction, 140
distribution, 16, 24, 74
dizygotic, 102
dizygotic twins, 102
DNA, 93, 99, 100
DNA damage, 100
dogs, 70
dominance, 4
dosing, 69
Down syndrome, 82
drawing, 31
drugs, viii, 91, 111, 112, 118
dwarfism, 82

156 Index

E

ectoderm, 73, 74
eczema, 99
edema, ix, 117, 132, 145, 146, 148, 149
education, 92, 94, 98, 138
egg, 93
Ehlers-Danlos syndrome, 76
electron, 63
electron microscopy, 63
embryogenesis, 61, 75
emergency, 147
employees, 103
encoding, 96
endothelium, viii, 74, 117, 124, 130
energy, 5
England, 60
enlargement, 64
enrollment, 125, 126
environmental factors, 91, 92, 102
environmental influences, 107
enzyme(s), 80, 91, 93, 97, 99
epidemiologic, 67, 90, 95, 103, 105
epidemiologic studies, 67, 95, 103
epidemiology, vii, viii, 59, 97, 98, 107
epinephrine, 115, 116, 120, 121
epithelial cells, 64, 86, 97, 103
epithelium, 67, 69, 72, 74, 99, 101, 108, 117
esotropia, 69
estrogen, 91
ethical issues, 139
ethnicity, 24
etiology, 70, 94, 108
Europe, 13
evidence, 28, 61, 67, 91, 92, 93, 95, 97, 105, 133, 148
evoked potential, 5
exclusion, 27
exercise, 138
exposure, 13, 64, 66, 67, 91, 92, 93, 94, 97, 101, 106, 107, 108
extracellular matrix, 97
extraction, 77, 83, 85, 141, 149

F

families, 70
family history, 76
feelings, 29
fiber(s), 62, 63, 64, 65, 67, 72, 75, 77, 81, 84, 96, 98
filters, 31, 92
financial, 139
fixation, 131, 133
flexibility, 103
fluctuations, 62
fluid, 63, 96, 98
fluttering, viii, 111, 112, 116
fMRI, 36
food, 94
Food and Drug Administration (FDA), 28
formation, 61, 62, 63, 64, 65, 66, 67, 68, 69, 79, 80, 82, 83, 84, 85, 86, 90, 91, 92, 93, 94, 96, 97, 107, 108
fragility, 71, 84
fraternal twins, 78
free radicals, 92, 96

G

gamma radiation, 93
gene expression, 97, 102
general anesthesia, 77
general surgery, 141
genes, 61, 70, 74, 78, 96, 97
genetic defect, 61
genetics, 61, 97, 102, 104, 105
geometry, 22, 23
Germany, 3, 10, 11, 16, 21, 23, 24
gestation, 74
glaucoma, vii, ix, 29, 69, 72, 75, 76, 77, 81, 82, 84, 85, 86, 104, 106, 109, 114, 125, 128, 134, 145, 146, 147, 148, 149, 150, 151
glucose, 67, 79, 80, 96
glutathione, 62, 97, 100, 108, 109
glycerol, 114, 118
glycosylation, 79

Index

grading, 28, 30, 31, 32, 107
gratings, 7, 8
growth, 82, 91, 96
growth factor, 91
guessing, 2, 9
guidance, 28
guidelines, 28, 112, 134

H

hair, 77
halos, 89
health, 92, 95, 146
health care, 146
heat shock protein, 97, 103
heavy metals, 95
height, 19
hemorrhage, 126, 149
hepatolenticular degeneration, 80
hepatomegaly, 80
herpes, 82, 99
herpes simplex, 82
herpes zoster, 99
heterogeneity, 102
history, 28, 84, 86, 100, 126, 146, 148
homeostasis, 97
human, 7, 17, 94, 97, 101, 102, 103, 105, 113, 139, 140, 151
hyperbaric oxygen therapy, 83, 106
hyperglycemia, 96
hypermature, ix, 64, 85, 87, 145, 146, 147, 148, 149, 150
hypertension, 68, 104
hypoplasia, 75
hypothesis, 93
hypotrichosis, 82

I

ideal, 10, 18, 19, 24
identification, 22, 25, 94, 97
idiopathic, 80, 99
illumination, 3, 11, 12, 31, 32
image(s), 15, 16, 18, 19, 20, 21, 22, 23, 24, 30, 31, 32
image analysis, 31, 32
imbalances, 91
immune response, 85
immunoglobulin, 84
improvements, 13
in utero, 74
in vitro, 103
incidence, viii, ix, 30, 61, 68, 69, 70, 75, 78, 91, 95, 104, 106, 107, 108, 109, 112, 116, 121, 124, 131, 133, 145
indentation, 73
India, 60, 106, 142
individuals, 60, 61, 63, 65, 66, 76, 77, 78, 92
induction, 139
infancy, 77
infants, 78
infection, 81, 90
inflammation, ix, 64, 68, 81, 84, 85, 126, 145, 149
informed consent, 125, 126
ingest, 85
inheritance, 78
inhibitor, 115, 149
initiation, 96, 109
injury(s), 65, 66, 67, 68, 84, 85, 93, 99, 103, 149
integrity, 63, 76, 84
internal consistency, 25, 28
internal environment, 97
intervention, 80
intraocular, vii, viii, ix, 1, 2, 18, 19, 20, 26, 64, 67, 68, 84, 85, 102, 104, 114, 124, 126, 127, 129, 131, 133, 145, 146, 149, 150
intraocular lenses, vii, 1, 2
intraocular pressure, ix, 68, 102, 114, 126, 127, 129, 133, 145, 146
intraoperative, vii, 114, 116, 119, 120, 121, 140
ion transport, 91
ionizing radiation, 64, 66, 93, 99, 105
Iowa, 143

iridotomy, 75, 86, 128, 133, 135
iris, vii, viii, 21, 23, 24, 67, 75, 76, 78, 79, 84, 86, 99, 111, 112, 113, 114, 115, 116, 117, 118, 119, 120, 121
iris prolapse, viii, 111, 116
iris syndrome, vii, viii, 111, 112, 119, 120, 121
iron, 67
irradiation, 91, 92, 93
irrigation, 112, 116, 118, 120, 147
ischemia, 99
isolation, 17
issues, ix, 5, 10, 137
Italy, 33

J

Japan, 21, 24, 30, 60, 112, 123, 125, 126, 134
jaundice, 80

K

Korea, 145

L

lamella, 66
languages, 6, 10
latency, 66
later life, 93
Latin America, 105
Latinos, 108
lead, 12, 15, 31, 66, 70, 94, 95, 96, 101, 113, 133, 138
leakage, ix, 145, 147, 148
leaks, 64
learning, vii, 13, 138, 139, 140, 141, 144
LED, 25
level of education, 92
light, 15, 16, 18, 19, 20, 21, 22, 23, 24, 30, 62, 63, 77, 83, 88, 89, 92, 93, 99, 101
light scattering, 30, 62, 63
lipid peroxidation, 100

liquefaction, ix, 64, 145, 146
liquids, 29
loci, 61, 97
locus, 78
longitudinal study, 70, 98, 103, 104
Luo, 102
lutein, 94
lymphocytes, 146
lysine, 78

M

macrophages, 85, 146, 147, 148, 149
macular degeneration, 104
magnitude, 7, 14, 18, 19, 21
Maillard reaction, 107
majority, 25, 61, 150
malnutrition, 80, 98
management, vii, ix, 86, 112, 115, 120, 133, 134, 135, 146, 150
manipulation, 23
Marfan syndrome, 75, 76, 77
mass, 62, 85, 98, 103
materials, 20, 31
matrix, 83, 97, 109
measurement(s), vii, 1, 2, 3, 4, 7, 8, 9, 11, 12, 13, 16, 17, 18, 19, 22, 23, 24, 31, 33, 126
media, 23
median, 138
mediation, 96
medical, viii, ix, 32, 59, 75, 86, 105, 111, 114, 138, 146, 149
medical history, viii, 111, 114
medication, 69, 112, 115, 121
medicine, 100, 113
mellitus, 79
membranes, 82
mental retardation, 75
meridian, 30
metabolic, 70, 79
metabolic disorder(s), 61, 70
metabolism, 77, 78, 79, 80, 82, 91, 96
metabolites, 63
metals, 91

Index

meter, 24
methodology, 7, 11
microscope, 126
microwave radiation, 67
microwaves, 93
migration, 64
miosis, 15, 64, 113, 116, 117
MIP, 96
mitosis, 99
mitral valve, 76
mitral valve prolapse, 76
models, 94
modifications, 63
molecular weight, 148, 151
molecules, 67
morbidity, viii, 59, 67, 140, 141
morphology, vii, viii, 59, 70, 100
mortality, 141
motivation, 10
muscle contraction, 11
muscles, 81
muscular tissue, 114
mutation(s), 70, 74, 76, 78, 96, 102, 105
myopia, 17, 63, 73, 77, 78, 98, 106

N

National Institutes of Health, 32
nearsightedness, 88
necrosis, 68, 86
neovascularization, 68
Nepal, 106, 151
nerve, ix, 75, 125, 126, 146
nervous system, 99
Netherlands, 117, 126
neuropathy, 69
niacin, 94
night driving, 26, 29
NSAIDs, 118
nuclei, 72, 81
nucleus, 62, 63, 64, 72, 80, 88, 90, 139, 146
null, 100
nutrition, 94
nutritional deficiencies, 92, 94
nystagmus, 75

O

obstruction, 148, 151
ocular diseases, 86
oil, 73, 80, 87
opacification, 15, 30, 31, 62, 63, 65, 66, 72, 73, 79, 80, 81, 83, 86, 88, 90, 99, 149
opacity, 32, 61, 62, 64, 71, 73, 74, 91, 95, 97, 99, 100
open angle glaucoma, ix, 145, 150
operations, 138
ophthalmologist, 62
ophthalmoscopy, 72
opportunities, 140
optic nerve, ix, 75, 125, 126, 146
optical systems, 23
organs, 83
osteomalacia, 82
osteonectin, 97
osteoporosis, 77
overlap, 22
oxalate, 146
oxidation, 90, 91, 92, 100, 107
oxidative damage, 92, 95
oxidative stress, 79, 84, 92, 96, 97, 103
oxygen, 83
ozone, 93
ozone layer, 93

P

paediatric patients, 23
pain, 85, 147, 148, 149
pairing, 127
paracentesis, 149
parathyroid, 80
parathyroid glands, 80
participants, 94
pathogenesis, viii, 59, 62
pathology, 87
pathways, 78, 97
perforation, 66, 132
phacoemulsification, vii, viii, ix, 85, 120, 124, 126, 127, 128, 129, 130, 131, 132,

133, 134, 135, 137, 138, 139, 140, 141, 142, 143, 144
phacolytic glaucoma, vii, ix, 85, 145, 146, 147, 148, 149, 150, 151
phenothiazines, 69
phenotypes, 70, 106
Philadelphia, 102, 105, 107, 150
phosphate, 80
photocells, 7
photographs, 21, 31, 100, 104, 147
photosensitizers, 92
pigmentation, 31, 62, 84
pilot study, 26
placebo, 100
plaque, 99
platform, 11
polar, 71, 72, 74, 75
polymorphisms, 109
polypeptide, 96
population, 23, 26, 29, 60, 67, 89, 94, 100, 101, 103, 104, 105, 106, 108, 113, 127, 133, 138, 146
portfolio, 33
posterior cortex, 63, 80
potassium, 62
precipitation, 63
pregnancy, 81, 90
preoperative precautions, viii, 111
preparation, 139
presbyopia, 9, 10, 11, 12, 13, 14, 26, 79
preservative, 116
prevention, 100
principles, 11
private practice, 138
prognosis, ix, 83, 145, 149
project, 71
prolapse, viii, 111, 112, 116, 149
proliferation, 91
prophylaxis, 121
protection, 97
protein oxidation, 63
protein synthesis, 97
proteins, viii, 59, 62, 73, 79, 84, 85, 87, 90, 92, 93, 96, 97, 99, 100, 148
proteolysis, 91

pseudophakia, 60, 101
psychometric properties, 27
psychotropic medications, 69
pterygium, 147
ptosis, 81
public health, 105
pyridoxine, 78

Q

quality of life, 142
questioning, viii, 111, 114
questionnaire, 26, 27, 28, 29, 33

R

race, 26
racial differences, 61
radial distance, 22
radiation, 65, 66, 67, 93, 99, 102, 105, 106, 108
radius, 22, 23
random assignment, 125
Rasch analysis, 26, 27, 29, 33
rating scale, 140
ray-tracing, 20
reaction time, 5
reactive oxygen, 92
reading, 3, 4, 5, 6, 9, 10, 11, 25, 77, 88, 89, 138, 139
realism, 10
reality, 143
receptors, 91
recession, 140
recognition, 3, 5
reconstruction, 18
recreational, 10
refractive index, 22, 24, 62, 79
refractive indices, 31
relaxation, 81, 113
reliability, 24
repair, 98
requirements, 67, 138, 139, 144
researchers, vii, 2, 19, 33

Index

resolution, 19, 126, 128
respiration, 96
response, 5, 8, 15, 16, 28, 29, 94, 112, 148
response time, 5
restoration, 14
retardation, 82
retina, 18, 19, 24, 67, 72, 75, 89
retinal detachment, 77, 78
retinitis, 86, 99
retinitis pigmentosa, 86, 99
retinopathy, 81
rheumatoid arthritis, 107
riboflavin, 94
rights, 147, 148
rings, viii, 3, 23, 111, 115, 117, 118
risk, vii, viii, 2, 59, 67, 70, 72, 77, 78, 79, 83, 87, 90, 91, 92, 93, 94, 95, 97, 98, 101, 103, 104, 105, 106, 107, 108, 114, 115, 116, 118, 142
risk factors, vii, viii, 59, 87, 90, 91, 95, 98, 104, 108, 142
RNA, 81
root, 18, 76
root-mean-square, 18
rotations, 21, 140
routes, 68
rubella, 70, 75, 81
rubella virus, 81
rural population, 106

S

safety, vii, viii, 124, 133
salmon, 108
sarcoidosis, 99
scatter, 18, 19, 20, 23, 24, 83, 62
science, 95
sclera, 24, 82
sclerosis, 62, 83, 87, 95, 98, 126, 128
scope, 30
segregation, 108
sensitivity, 7, 8, 9, 17
sex, 127
shape, 16, 24, 25, 73, 75, 81, 118
shock, 68, 97

showing, 92, 133
side effects, 118
signal transduction, 102
signs, 63, 65, 66, 115, 116, 117, 148, 150
single test, 33
skin, 140
slit lamp, 31, 64, 65, 75, 108, 126
slit lamp examination, 126
smoking, 92, 94, 95, 97, 98, 103, 108
smooth muscle, 113
social activities, 25
socioeconomic status, 92, 94
sodium, 62, 97
software, 4, 7, 18, 21, 22, 30, 31, 32
solution, 112, 116, 118
Spain, 18
spatial frequency, 7, 19
spatial location, 25
species, 92
sphincter, 115
stability, 20, 21
statin, 70
statistics, 60, 126
steroids, ix, 68, 91, 145, 149
stimulation, 16
stimulus, 16
strabismus, 82
stress, 92, 96, 97, 106, 108
stretching, 118
stroma, 112, 115
structural protein, 97
structure, 24, 63, 140
style(s), 20, 119
subluxation, 65, 76, 77, 84
success rate, 60
sulfate, 120
Sun, 105, 106, 107, 109
supplementation, 100
surgical removal, 86, 150
surgical technique, 30
suture, 131
sutureless, vii, 124, 125, 133
swelling, 64, 98
Switzerland, 3

symptoms, 24, 26, 28, 72, 80, 89, 113, 114, 120, 148
syndrome, vii, viii, 70, 73, 74, 75, 76, 77, 81, 82, 83, 84, 90, 96, 99, 107, 109, 111, 112, 118, 119, 120, 121, 128
synthesis, 97
syphilis, 99

T

tamoxifen, 70, 91
target, 3, 4, 7, 12, 15, 16, 24, 25, 33
techniques, vii, ix, 1, 2, 17, 21, 30, 32, 33, 134, 137, 139, 140, 142
technology, 32, 138
temperature, 99
tension, 83
testing, 4, 7, 9, 143
texture, 31
therapy, 69, 78, 83, 85, 101, 107, 113, 124, 149
thinning, 74
thorax, 66
threshold level, 13
thromboangiitis obliterans, 86
thyroid, 80
tissue, 79
tobacco, 95
tobacco smoke, 95
tonometry, 126
topical steroids, ix, 145, 149
toxic effect, 92
toxicity, 95
toxoplasmosis, 82, 99
trabecular meshwork, ix, 67, 84, 85, 145, 148
trainees, 140, 142
training, ix, 137, 139, 140, 143, 144
training programs, 139
traits, 25
trajectory, 23
transcription, 74, 75, 99
transcription factors, 74
transformation, 96
transforming growth factor (TGF), 84
translation, 29
transmission, 67, 68
transparency, 31, 32, 62
transport, 97
trauma, 20, 64, 65, 98, 114, 148
treatment, vii, ix, 5, 68, 69, 71, 75, 83, 85, 86, 93, 113, 114, 115, 133, 145, 149
trial, 100, 127, 135
trisomy 21, 82
tuberculosis, 99
tumor, 75
Turkey, 112
type 1 diabetes, 79

U

ultrasonography, 126
ultrasound, 16
uniform, 25
united, 3, 60, 67, 91, 101, 120, 138, 139, 140, 143, 146
United Kingdom (UK), 1, 3, 4, 112, 117, 118, 120, 140, 143
United States (USA), 3, 60, 67, 91, 101, 112, 125, 138, 139, 140, 146
universities, 138
urban, 100
urinary retention, 115, 118
urinary tract, 113, 114, 120
urine, 80
US Department of Health and Human Services, 28
UV light, 91, 93
UV radiation, 67, 93, 107
uveitis, 82, 84, 85, 99, 103, 146, 151

V

validation, 25, 28
variables, 127
variations, 3, 19, 20, 22, 31, 76, 77, 92, 119
vascular diseases, 113
vasculature, 78
vesicle, 74

vessels, 79
videos, 138
viscosity, 117
vision, 4, 5, 6, 9, 10, 11, 12, 13, 14, 23, 26, 28, 29, 60, 62, 64, 65, 68, 71, 72, 76, 85, 86, 88, 89, 100, 103, 105, 142, 147, 149
visual acuity, vii, viii, 3, 5, 6, 59, 71, 72, 77, 104, 124, 126, 127, 128, 146
visualization, 119, 149
vitamin A, 94
vitamin B6, 78
vitamin C, 94, 100, 106
vitamin E, 94
vitamin supplementation, 78
vitamins, 93, 94, 100
vitrectomy, vii, viii, 77, 83, 124, 125, 127, 128, 129, 130, 131, 132, 133, 134
volunteers, 51
vomiting, 147

W

water, 63, 89, 100, 114
weakness, 81, 84
workers, 11, 12, 26, 31, 93, 99
workplace, 103
World Health Organization (WHO), 60
worldwide, vii, 59, 60

X

x-rays, 93, 99

Y

yield, 4
young people, 79